Antonio M. Esquinas
Editor

High-Frequency Chest Wall Oscillation Therapy in Critically Ill Patients

A Rational Approach

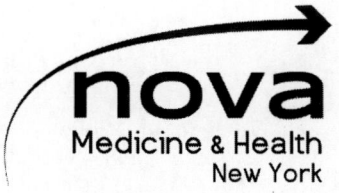

Copyright © 2025 by Nova Science Publishers, Inc.
DOI: https://doi.org/10.52305/QXLQ7155

All rights reserved. No part of this book may be reproduced, stored in a retrieval system or transmitted in any form or by any means: electronic, electrostatic, magnetic, tape, mechanical photocopying, recording or otherwise without the written permission of the Publisher.

We have partnered with Copyright Clearance Center to make it easy for you to obtain permissions to reuse content from this publication. Simply navigate to this publication's page on Nova's website and locate the "Get Permission" button below the title description. This button is linked directly to the title's permission page on copyright.com. Alternatively, you can visit copyright.com and search by title, ISBN, or ISSN.

For further questions about using the service on copyright.com, please contact:
Copyright Clearance Center
Phone: +1-(978) 750-8400   Fax: +1-(978) 750-4470   E-mail: info@copyright.com

NOTICE TO THE READER

The Publisher has taken reasonable care in the preparation of this book, but makes no expressed or implied warranty of any kind and assumes no responsibility for any errors or omissions. No liability is assumed for incidental or consequential damages in connection with or arising out of information contained in this book. The Publisher shall not be liable for any special, consequential, or exemplary damages resulting, in whole or in part, from the readers' use of, or reliance upon, this material. Any parts of this book based on government reports are so indicated and copyright is claimed for those parts to the extent applicable to compilations of such works.

Independent verification should be sought for any data, advice or recommendations contained in this book. In addition, no responsibility is assumed by the Publisher for any injury and/or damage to persons or property arising from any methods, products, instructions, ideas or otherwise contained in this publication.

This publication is designed to provide accurate and authoritative information with regard to the subject matter covered herein. It is sold with the clear understanding that the Publisher is not engaged in rendering legal or any other professional services. If legal or any other expert assistance is required, the services of a competent person should be sought. FROM A DECLARATION OF PARTICIPANTS JOINTLY ADOPTED BY A COMMITTEE OF THE AMERICAN BAR ASSOCIATION AND A COMMITTEE OF PUBLISHERS.

Additional color graphics may be available in the e-book version of this book.

Library of Congress Cataloging-in-Publication Data

ISBN: 979-8-89530-264-4 (Softcover)
ISBN: 979-8-89530-403-7 (eBook)

Published by Nova Science Publishers, Inc. † New York

Contents

Chapter 1	The History of High-Frequency Chest Wall Oscillatory Therapy..........1 Kıvanç Terzi	
Chapter 2	High-Frequency Chest Wall Oscillation: Vibration and Oscillation Effects on the Respiratory System..........7 Salvatore Musella, Elena Sciarrillo and Antonio M. Esquinas	
Chapter 3	High-Frequency Chest Wall Oscillation Waveforms: Clinical Implications..........15 Kumari Sulochana, Kishore Kumar, George Savio Chellam and Antonio M. Esquinas	
Chapter 4	High-Frequency Chest Wall Oscillation: Equipment..........29 Mostafa Elshazly and Ahmed Tantawy	
Chapter 5	High-Frequency Chest Wall Oscillation: Setting Pressure and Frequency..........37 Mohamad F. El-Khatib	
Chapter 6	High-Frequency Chest Wall Oscillation: Clinical Monitoring..........43 Mostafa Elshazly and Mohamed Kamal Hasswa	
Chapter 7	How to Evaluate High-Frequency Chest Wall Oscillation in Mechanical Ventilation..........51 Cátia Pimentel	

Contents

Chapter 8 High-Frequency Chest Wall Oscillation Therapy in the Critically Ill: Summary and Key Practical Approaches 63
Ahmad Mohammad Alessa
and Antonio M. Esquinas

Chapter 9 High-Frequency Chest Wall Oscillation and Nasal High Flow Oxygen 75
Francisco Neri

Chapter 10 Weaning from Mechanical Ventilation and Pulmonary Rehabilitation 81
Berkan Basançelebi

Chapter 11 High-Frequency Chest Wall Oscillation in Extubation Respiratory Failure 93
Inês Martinho Santos Jorge

Chapter 12 High-Frequency Chest Wall Oscillation in Chronic Obstructive Pulmonary Disorder 101
Salvatore Notaro, Vincezo Capaldo,
Andrea Imparato and Eugenio Piscitelli

Chapter 13 High-Frequency Chest Wall Oscillation in Neuromuscular Pulmonary Disorders 121
Elvia Giovanna Battaglia, Elena Compalati,
Salvatore Sciurello, Giuseppe Russo
and Paolo Innocente Banfi

Chapter 14 High-Frequency Chest Wall Oscillation for Ventilator-Associated Pneumonia 135
Hılal Sıpahıoglu

Chapter 15 High-Frequency Chest Wall Oscillation for Cystic Fibrosis Exacerbations in Pediatrics 145
Mariana Celiz Alonso

Chapter 16 High-Frequency Chest Wall Oscillation Applications for Non-Cystic Fibrosis Children 155
Merve Erdem and Selman Kesici

About the Editor 165

Index 167

Chapter 1

The History of High-Frequency Chest Wall Oscillatory Therapy

Kıvanç Terzi[*], MD
Ağrı Training and Research Hospital,
Department of Pediatric Intensive Care, Ağrı, Turkey

Abstract

High-Frequency Chest Wall Oscillation (HFCWO) therapy has evolved since its initial use in treating cystic fibrosis. This comprehensive review examines the history, mechanisms, and effects of HFCWO on respiratory health by focusing on critical studies across various diseases and patient populations. Early studies demonstrated the effectiveness of HFCWO in enhancing tracheal mucus clearance and supporting respiratory functions in conditions such as COPD. Subsequent research expanded its use to cystic fibrosis, which proved to be as effective as traditional therapies for mucus clearance. In the early 2000s, HFCWO was explored in neurological diseases, showing improved lung function and symptom reduction. Later studies indicated the benefits of HFCWO in treating acute respiratory ailments and post-lung transplant care, highlighting its role in decreasing pain and improving patient preferences compared to chest physiotherapy. Further research confirmed the effectiveness of HFCWO in pediatric care, particularly in treating pneumonia and critical care settings, by improving oxygenation and lung compliance. Overall, HFCWO has expanded its applications beyond cystic fibrosis, demonstrating significant potential in enhancing respiratory therapy and improving patient outcomes across respiratory conditions.

---

[*] Corresponding Author's Email: kvnctrz@gmail.com.

In: High-frequency Chest Wall Oscillation Therapy in Critical Ill Patients
Editor: Antonio M. Esquinas
ISBN: 979-8-89530-264-4
© 2025 Nova Science Publishers, Inc.

Keywords: high-frequency, oscillation, respiratory therapy, mucus clearance

Introduction

This chapter provides a comprehensive evaluation of the history of HFCWO. It examines the evolution, mechanism, and effects of HFCWO on respiratory health. The review focuses on critical studies on the use of HFCWO in various diseases and patient populations, paying particular attention to the timing of these studies, thus providing a thorough assessment of the history of HFCWO [1].

Recent Findings

HFCWO is widely used for airway clearance in various respiratory conditions, including cystic fibrosis, bronchiectasis, neuromuscular disorders, and chronic obstructive pulmonary disease (COPD) [1]. The technique involves applying high-velocity, low-amplitude oscillatory airflows through a pneumatic vest worn over the thorax, which helps clear mucus from the airways [2].

In the first-ever use of HFCWO, King et al. conducted an experimental study on anesthetized dogs. They demonstrated that the tracheal mucus clearance rate (TMCR) significantly increased, especially within the frequency range of 11 to 15 Hz, through the application of High-Frequency Chest Wall Compression (HFCWC) using a thoracic cuff to generate oscillatory tidal volumes between 3 Hz and 17 Hz, as determined by direct observation via a fiberoptic bronchoscope [3]. In 1987, it was found in patients with chronic obstructive pulmonary disease (COPD) that the application of 5 Hz HFCWO, used only during the expiratory phase to prevent discomfort, significantly altered respiratory frequency and tidal volume. Researchers demonstrated that HFCWO improved arterial gas exchange and supported inspiratory muscle function in COPD patients [2]. Following the use of HFCWO in patients with COPD, studies began to explore the application of HFCWO in patients with cystic fibrosis. Kluft and colleagues conducted a study in 1996 comparing standard chest physical therapy and postural drainage (CPT/PD) and HFCWO in stable cystic fibrosis (CF) patients. The results showed that HFCWO was at least as effective as manual CPT/PD in clearing airway secretions in CF patients, as it facilitated the expectoration of more sputum according to wet and dry weight measurements compared to CPT/PD [4].

Before 2005, there were no studies on using HFCWO outside cystic fibrosis. However, in 2005, a study was published regarding using HFCWO in neurological diseases. In the study conducted by Giarraffa and colleagues, using HFCWO in patients with familial dysautonomia was observed to improve lung function indicators such as oxygen saturation, Forced Vital Capacity (FVC), and Peak Expiratory Flow Rate (PEFR) and significantly reduce the number of hospitalizations and antibiotic usage [5]. A second study, published in 2006, also focused on using HFCWO in neurological diseases. Lange and colleagues observed in their study that applying HFCWO in patients with Amyotrophic Lateral Sclerosis (ALS) reduced symptoms of dyspnea and, in patients with limited respiratory function, slowed the decline in FVC, thereby alleviating fatigue. The study findings indicate that HFCWO therapy was generally well-tolerated by patients and considered therapeutically beneficial by the majority [6].

In 2011, a randomized, multi-center clinical trial conducted by Mahajan and colleagues demonstrated that the early use of HFCWO in adults hospitalized for acute asthma or COPD significantly improved dyspnea, with high patient adherence and satisfaction, indicating good tolerability. The study highlights the necessity for further research to comprehensively assess the impact of HFCWO on in-hospital and post-discharge outcomes [7]. It also demonstrated that clinicians could use HFCWO to treat acute exacerbations of obstructive lung diseases. A study conducted in 2013 compared the effects of HFCWO and chest physiotherapy on pain and patient preferences in post-lung transplant patients, revealing that HFCWO, especially in bilateral transplant recipients, led to more significant decreases in pain scores and was more preferred compared to chest physiotherapy. The study emphasizes that HFCWO may be a practical and feasible alternative to chest physiotherapy in post-lung transplant care [8]. This study demonstrated that using HFCWO is beneficial for a new indication.

Nicolini and colleagues conducted a study that evaluated HFCWO for use in lung disease, specifically in cases of chronic hypersecretion. This study compared CPT and HFCWO in patients with bronchiectasis and revealed that HFCWO significantly improved blood inflammation parameters, lung function, and dyspnea compared to CPT. The results have established HFCWO as a primary treatment method within chest physiotherapy for patients with chronic hypersecretory disease [9].

Usenko and colleagues conducted a study showing that HFCWO can be used in children for cystic fibrosis and other restrictive lung diseases [10]. This study demonstrated the positive effects of HFCWO on main clinical symptoms like cough severity and efficiency, as well as moist rales, treating community-acquired pneumonia (CAP) in children. It also showed improvements in mucociliary clearance (MCC) functions and overall healing of the bronchopulmonary system. The reduction in cough severity confirmed the effectiveness of HFCWO in treating CAP, the amount of sputum, and the decrease in rales in the lungs of children. These findings opened the way for its use in children diagnosed with pneumonia [10].

A randomized controlled study conducted by Ge and colleagues showed that HFCWO improves oxygenation and static lung compliance in critically ill patients admitted to the intensive care unit. The study also revealed that HFCWO effectively increases pulmonary surfactant proteins in the airways and reduces their transition from the blood to the airways [11].

Conclusion

Initially used in patients with cystic fibrosis, HFCWO has, over time, expanded its application to a broader spectrum of diseases, including COPD, bronchiectasis, neuromuscular disorders, and even acute respiratory ailments [12]. Studies have shown that HFCWO enhances mucus clearance, improves respiratory functions, reduces hospitalization durations, and increases treatment adherence and patient satisfaction [13]. This therapy has also emerged as an effective alternative in pediatric and post-lung transplant care. The expanding applications of HFCWO and its positive outcomes underscore its significance in respiratory treatments and provide an encouraging foundation for further.

Key Messages

1. Initially tested on animals, HFCWO was first applied to humans in the 1980s, showing effectiveness in COPD patients. This initial success marked the beginning of its use in respiratory care.

2. By 1996, HFCWO was compared with standard treatments in cystic fibrosis, proving to be equally effective. This comparison expanded its application beyond its initial uses.
3. In 2005, studies demonstrated the benefits of HFCWO in neurological conditions like familial dysautonomia and ALS, broadening its therapeutic scope.
4. Throughout the 2010s, HFCWO emerged as a practical and versatile option for patients with acute respiratory distress and post-lung transplant, instilling confidence in its adaptability to new clinical settings.

References

[1] McIlwaine, M. P., N. Alarie, G. F. Davidson, L. C. Lands, F. Ratjen, R. Milner, B. Owen, J. L. Agnew. Long-term multicentre randomised controlled study of high-frequency chest wall oscillation versus positive expiratory pressure mask in cystic fibrosis. *Thorax* 2013: 68, no. 8 746-751.

[2] Piquet, J., L. Brochard, D. Isabey, H. de Cremoux, H. K. Chang, J. Bignon, ve A. Harf. High-frequency chest wall oscillation in patients with chronic air-flow obstruction. *The American Review of Respiratory Disease* 1987: 136, no. 6 1355-1359.

[3] King, M., D. M. Phillips, D. Gross, V. Vartian, H. K. Chang, ve A. Zidulka. Enhanced tracheal mucus clearance with high-frequency chest wall compression. *The American Review of Respiratory Disease* 1983; 128, no. 3: 511-515.

[4] Kluft, J., L. Beker, M. Castagnino, J. Gaiser, H. Chaney, ve R. J. Fink. A comparison of bronchial drainage treatments in cystic fibrosis. *Pediatric Pulmonology* 1996; 22, no. 4: 271-274.

[5] Giarraffa, P., K. I. Berger, A. A. Chaikin, F. B. Axelrod, C. Davey, ve B. Becker. Assessing efficacy of high-frequency chest wall oscillation in patients with familial dysautonomia. *Chest* 2005; 128, no. 5: 3377-3381.

[6] Lange, D. J., N. Lechtzin, C. Davey, W. David, T. Heiman-Patterson, D. Gelinas, B. Becker, H. Mitsumoto. HFCWO Study Group. High-frequency chest wall oscillation in ALS: an exploratory randomized, controlled trial. *Neurology* 2006; 67, no. 6: 991-997.

[7] Mahajan, A. K., G. B. Diette, U. Hatipoğlu, A. Bilderback, A. Ridge, V. W. Harris, V. Dalapathi, S. Badlani, S. Lewis, J. T. Charbeneau, E. T. Naureckas, ve J. A. Krishnan. High-frequency chest wall oscillation for asthma and chronic obstructive pulmonary disease exacerbations: a randomized sham-controlled clinical trial. *Respiratory Research* 2011; 12, no. 1: 120.

[8] Esguerra-Gonzalez, A., M. Ilagan-Honorio, S. Fraschilla, P. Kehoe, A. J. Lee, T. Marcarian, K. Mayol-Ngo, P. S. Miller, J. Onga, B. Rodman, D. Ross, S. Sommer, S. Takayanagi, J. Toyama, F. Villamor, S. S. Weigt, ve A. Gawlinski. CNE article:

pain after lung transplant: high-frequency chest wall oscillation vs chest physiotherapy. *American Journal of Critical Care: An Official Publication, American Association of Critical-Care Nurses* 2013; 22, no. 2: 115-124.
[9] Nicolini, A., F. Cardini, N. Landucci, S. Lanata, M. Ferrari-Bravo, ve C. Barlascini. Effectiveness of treatment with high-frequency chest wall oscillation in patients with bronchiectasis. *BMC Pulmonary Medicine* (2013) 13: 21.
[10] Usenko, D. V., ve M. L. Aryayev. Effect of high-frequency chest wall oscillation on clinical indices of community-acquired pneumonia in children. Wiadomości Lekarskie (Warsaw, Poland: 1960) 2022; 75, no. 12: 3004-3009.
[11] Ge, J., Y. Ye, Y. Tan, F. Liu, Y. Jiang, ve J. Lu. High-frequency chest wall oscillation multiple times daily can better reduce the loss of pulmonary surfactant and improve lung compliance in mechanically ventilated patients. Heart & Lung: *The Journal of Critical Care* 2023; 61: 114-119.
[12] Longhini, F., A. Bruni, E. Garofalo, C. Ronco, A. Gusmano, G. Cammarota, L. Pasin, P. Frigerio, D. Chiumello, ve P. Navalesi. Chest physiotherapy improves lung aeration in hypersecretive critically ill patients: a pilot randomized physiological study. *Critical Care (London, England)* 2020; 24, no. 1 479.
[13] Leemans, G., D. Belmans, C. Van Holsbeke, B. Becker, D. Vissers, K. Ides, S. Verhulst, ve K. Van Hoorenbeeck. The effectiveness of a mobile high-frequency chest wall oscillation (HFCWO) device for airway clearance. *Pediatric Pulmonology* 2020 ;55, no. 8: 1984-1992.

Chapter 2

High-Frequency Chest Wall Oscillation: Vibration and Oscillation Effects on the Respiratory System

Salvatore Musella[1,*], RT
Elena Sciarrillo[1], RT
and Antonio M. Esquinas[2], MD, PhD, FCCP, FNIV

[1]Physiopathology and Pulmonary Rehabilitation, Monaldi Hospital, Naples, Italy
[2]Intensive Care Unit; Hospital Morales Meseguer. Murcia, Spain

Abstract

Most airway clearance techniques, use external or internal vibrations and oscillations in order to increase air-mucus interaction, promote the mucociliary escalator and ease the movement of secretions from the distal to the proximal airways, in pathological conditions. This chapter analyzes some types of vibrations and oscillations and their effects on the respiratory system in normal and in pathological conditions.

Keywords: vibration, oscillation, respiratory system, mucus movement, airway clearance

---

* Corresponding Author's Email: salvatoremusella@outlook.com.

In: High-frequency Chest Wall Oscillation Therapy in Critical Ill Patients
Editor: Antonio M. Esquinas
ISBN: 979-8-89530-264-4
© 2025 Nova Science Publishers, Inc.

Introduction

Mucociliary transport is a defense mechanism that protects the pulmonary system from the harmful effects of foreign inhaled substances [1]. It is driven by ciliated cells and constitutes the predominant clearance mechanism in healthy subjects; however, it also plays a pivotal role in pathological conditions where ciliary permeability is impaired and mucociliary transport is inadequate. It can be altered by changes in the rheological properties of the mucus and is dependent on proper cilia function [1].

Several factors can interfere with the body's natural defense mechanism, making it difficult to mobilize the mucus in the direction of the bigger airways. Various methods and techniques have been developed over the years to facilitate and support the drainage of secretory products.

Airway clearance therapy facilitates the mobilization of mucus from the distal airways to the proximal respiratory tract.

Some mechanical and manual airway clearance techniques use vibrations and oscillations to increase air-mucus interaction and promote the movement of secretions from the distal to the proximal airways where this does not normally occur.

The alveolar air/tissue interface is crucial for gas exchanges. When the tissue is compressed, the air flows from the tissue into the airway tree; when the tissue expands, the air flows from the tree into the tissue. Airflow through the tree is maintained and air is exchanged with the surrounding air through the first-generation airway, which mimics the trachea, with all terminal branches connected to the tissue. The air flow is distributed in the tree depending on the air pressure distribution resulting from the hydrodynamic resistances of the paths between the terminal branches and between the terminal branches and the trachea. The air pressure at the end of the terminal branches is felt by the tissue and in turn influences its tendency to compress or expand [1].

Chest vibrations are a unique biomechanical process in which stresses and strains occur in the unique biphasic medium of the lung with two media: compressible low-density gas and incompressible high-density soft tissue. This special nature of the media causes specific acoustic and other physical phenomena in the lungs and chest.

Various types of chest wall vibrations have been observed in the human chest wall and lungs [2].

Spontaneous vibrations in the lungs and chest wall at frequencies other than the respiratory rate occur as a result of breathing in the form of breath sounds or as a result of non-breathing mechanical activity in the chest (e.g., heartbeat). Breathing produces breath sounds by several mechanisms, including the production of sounds by vortices, by flattening and by tension relaxation in the lung parenchyma [3]. Vortices occur in transitional and turbulent flows in the airways. A large flow in a channel with an abrupt change in the channel profile can cause flow separation, i.e., a divergence of neighboring streamlines. Flow separation in a 3-dimensional structure such as airways creates vortices. Vortices can occur in the branches of the airways during both exhalation and inhalation [4]. The pressure fluctuations in the vortices lead to vibrations in the airways, the lung tissue and the chest wall, i.e., breathing noises. The vertebrae are the main source of normal lung sounds and some other breath sounds [5].

The duration of the forced expiratory tracheal sounds increases with gas density, which is further evidence that vortices are the main cause of the sounds [6].

Forced vibrations are the vibrations of the lung and chest wall tissue caused by external vibrations acting on the lung tissue. External vibrations are forced on the respiratory system for diagnostic and therapeutic purposes. To improve mucus clearance, therapists apply vibrations to the airways and/or the chest wall. Therapeutic vibrations are usually stronger than diagnostic vibrations.

Mechanical vibrations of the chest wall have been shown to alter the sensation of breathing [7]. There are several mechanisms by which intercostal vibration could influence "shortness of breath": One of the hypotheses is that vibration may stimulate afferent activity of the muscles of the chest wall (i.e., muscle spindles and/or Golgi tendon organs), as occurs in animals. These changes in spontaneous respiratory drive can lead to changes in the sensation of breathing. Chest wall vibration reduces dyspnea induced by a combination of hypercarbia and extrinsic or intrinsic load, as in patients with chronic obstructive pulmonary disease.

There is an alternative mechanism by which vibrations can influence breathing control if vibration on the chest wall reaches the airways, it is possible that the effects on sensation are mediated by lung receptors [7]. The effects of pulmonary receptor afferents on breathing control are well documented, but little is known about how these receptors might respond to vibration. Vibration of the chest wall may be the cause of the rapid oscillations of the lung parenchyma and airways.

A significant increase in peak expiratory flow was only observed when chest wall vibrations were used optimally or early in the breath cycle [8]. Late chest wall vibrations were not associated with an increase in absolute expiratory airflow. This suggests that chest wall vibrations must be used early or just before expiration to generate sufficient expiratory flow to be effective. However, early chest wall vibrations were also associated with a significant increase in peak inspiratory flow. Kazakia and Rivlin et al. investigated the effects of longitudinal, transverse and rotational vibrations and their combination on the non-Newtonian fluid flow in a pipe in various analytical studies [9]. They showed that if the viscosity of the fluid decreases by increasing the shear rate, the outflow rate of the non-Newtonian fluid can increase with the vibration frequency and amplitude. The fluid flow in their work is assumed to be laminar.

Flow oscillation is an effective method of removing mucus from the airways by various mechanisms:

1. It alters the viscoelasticity of mucus and reduces its stickiness and viscosity
2. It promotes gas-liquid interactions in the airways
3. It creates larger expiratory flow peaks than inspiratory flow peaks, shifting secretions from the peripheral to the proximal airways
4. It increases ciliary activity.

Chang et al. hypothesized that a mouthward bias of air velocity in asymmetric oscillatory flow would lead to a net inward movement of the mucosa [10].

This is related to the shear stress at the air-mucus interface and the velocity profiles of the airflow during the oscillatory flow.

Sputum is a viscoelastic medium that, in order to be cleared from the airways, should be subjected to fairly high shear stresses that exceed a threshold of fluidity. The compression impulses produce transient peaks of airflow peaks in the airways, directed cephalad. The airflow in the lungs is similar to that which occurs during a huffing maneuver, with the associated mucus shear force and a possible change in the physical properties of the mucus [11]. Some experiments have presented data indicating a reduction in the viscosity of mucus as a result of shear forces at the air-mucus interface [12]. It was found that the changes in the physical properties of mucus depend on the shear forces between air and mucus during coughing and on the time between coughs. The first cough leads to a decrease in mucus viscosity as a result of these shear forces, so that successive coughs move a less viscous mucus. It has also been found that the time between coughs is important.

The longer the time between coughs, the more the mucus can return to its original structure with increasing viscosity. The decrease in the viscoelastic modulus of mucus after oscillations could classically be explained by a decrease in the number of cross-links and entanglements of the macromolecules responsible for this rheological parameter. The entanglements may also depend on the degree of hydration of the gel-like polymers. In some experiments, however, the controls did not show a significant change in either spinnability or viscoelasticity, which even went insignificantly in the opposite direction for viscoelasticity. Burton et al. show that oscillating pressure stress increases ATP release on the surface of the airways. Increased ATP concentration at the airway surface results in a shift in the pattern of ion transport from absorption to secretion, via activation of apical purinoreceptors, leading to fluid secretion and acceleration of mucociliary clearance. In this way, the normal lung can respond to stress-inducing stimuli in the intrapulmonary airways by stimulating secretion and accelerating clearance, thereby promoting lung health [13]. Brunengo et al. show that tension due to airway wall vibration predominates in the upper part of the tree, while tension due to air-mucus interactions predominates in the deep parts of the tree [1]. We show that the frequencies from 3 Hz to 15 Hz maximize the airflow within the tree and thus the air–mucus interactions. This range corresponds to the typical operating frequencies used empirically in external chest wall vibrations. External chest oscillations have been shown to reduce end-expiratory lung volume in patients with airway disease to up to 50% of functional residual capacity due to the increased stress on the chest wall [14]. External shaking is associated with a drastic reduction in nitric oxide concentrations. Sisson et al. speculate that external mechanical shaking improves mucus clearance by stimulating calcium release from airway epithelial cells, leading to calmodulin activation of endothelial nitric oxide synthase, which in turn causes nitric oxide production in airway epithelial cells [15]. External mechanical vibrations influence the movement of the air in peripheral pulmonary tract [16].

Pendelluft is the movement of air between adjacent lung units (the functional unit of gas exchange consisting of structures containing alveoli located distal to the end of the terminal bronchiole) that have different time constants. The time constant for a lung is defined as the time it takes for a lung to empty or fill and is equal to the product of its resistance to airflow and its compliance. The air movement in the lungs is therefore dependent on the diameter of the airways and the elasticity of the tissue. Time constants are slow when lung units have low distensibility and high airway resistance. Parallel lung units, present in the same lung region, normally fill and empty at about the same rates. However, in obstructive lung disease, parallel lung units frequently fill and empty at different rates. During external chest wall shaking, *pendelluft* may increase the recirculation of air, thereby increasing alveolar ventilation for previously closed or under ventilated lung units. The results are improvements in gas mixing and homogenization of expired gas concentrations from these neighboring lung units [15, 16].

Conclusion

Both vibrations and oscillations significantly affect mucociliary clearance by favoring the interaction between airflow and secretions and influencing the rheological properties of mucus, especially in pathological situations: they reduce the density of mucus and increase air-mucus interaction within the airways. This means that these physical phenomena are widely used in electromedical devices dedicated to the management of patients with bronchial hypersecretion.

Key Messages

1. Some mechanical and manual airway clearance techniques use external or internal vibration and oscillation to increase air-mucus interaction, facilitate mucociliary escalator activity, and promote the movement of secretions from the distal to the proximal airways.
2. The compression impulses produce transient peaks of airflow peaks in the airways, directed cephalad, similar to that which occurs during a huffing maneuver, with the associated mucus shear force and a possible change in the physical properties of the mucus.
3. Flow oscillation alters the viscoelasticity of mucus and reduces its stickiness and viscosity, promotes gas-liquid interactions in the airways, creates larger expiratory flow peaks than inspiratory flow peaks, shifting secretions from the peripheral to the proximal airways and increases ciliary activity.
4. During external chest wall shaking, pendelluft may increase the recirculation of air, thereby increasing alveolar ventilation. The

results are improvements in gas mixing and homogenization of expired gas concentrations from these neighboring lung units.

References

[1] Brunengo M, Mitchell BR, Nicolini A, Rousselet B, Mauroy B. Optimal efficiency of high-frequency chest wall oscillations and links with resistance and compliance in a model of the lung. *Physics of Fluids* 2021; 33(12):121909.
[2] D'yachenko AI. Biophysics of chest vibrations. *J Apl Theol* 2017; 1, 14–19.
[3] Pasterkamp H, Kraman S, Wodicka G. Respiratory Sounds. Advances beyond the stethoscope. *Am J Respir Crit Care Med* 1997; 156 (3):974–987.
[4] Hardin JC, Patterson JLJr. Monitoring the state of the human airways by analysis of respiratory sound. *Acta Astronautica* 1979; 6(9):1137–1151.
[5] Bohadana A, Izbicki G, Kraman S. Fundamentals of Lung Auscultation. *N Engl J Med* 2014; 370:744-751.
[6] D'yachenko AI, Korenbaum VI, Kir'yanova EV, Pochekutova IA, Shulagin YA, Osipova AA. Effect of Respiratory Gases Composition on Duration of Forced Expiratory Tracheal Noises. In: Proceed. 3-rd Russian-Bavarian Conf; 2007 July 2-3; Erlangen, Bavaria: Biomed. Eng, 2007. p. 204-206.
[7] Binks AP, Bloch-Salisbury E, Banzett RB, Schwartzstein RM. Oscillation of the lung by chest-wall vibration. *Respir Physiol* 2001; 126(3):245-9.
[8] Shannon H, Stiger R, Gregson RK, Stocks J, Main E. Effect of chest wall vibration timing on peak expiratory flow and inspiratory pressure in a mechanically ventilated lung model. *Physiotherapy* 2010; 96(4):344-9.
[9] Kazakia JY, Rivlin RS. The influence of vibration on Poiseuille flow of a non-Newtonian fluid. *I Rheol Acta* 1979; 2:244–55.
[10] Chang HK, Weber ME, King M. Mucus transport by high-frequency nonsymmetrical oscillatory airflow. *Journal of Applied Physiology* 1988; 65(3), 1203–1209.
[11] Hansen LG, Warwick WJ, Hansen KL. Mucus transport mechanisms in relation to the effect of high-frequency chest compression (HFCC) on mucus clearance. *Pediatr Pulmonol* 1994; 17: 113-118.
[12] Zahm JM, King M, Duvivier C, Pierrot D, Girod S, Puchelle E. Role of simulated repetitive coughing in mucus clearance. *Eur Respir J* 1991; 4(3):311-5.
[13] Button B, Picher M, Boucher RC. Differential effects of cyclic and constant stress on ATP release and mucociliary transport by human airway epithelia. *J Physiol* 2007; 580(Pt. 2):577-92.
[14] Jones RL, Lester RT, Brown NE. Effects of high-frequency chest compression on respiratory system mechanics in normal subjects and cystic fibrosis patients. *Can Respir J* 1995; 2:40-6.
[15] Sisson JH, Wyatt TA, Pavlik JA, Sarna PS, Murphy PJ. Vest Chest Physiotherapy Airway Clearance is Associated with Nitric Oxide Metabolism. *Pulm Med* 2013; 2013:291375.

[16] Darbee JC, Kanga JF, Ohtake PJ. Physiologic evidence for high-frequency chest wall oscillation and positive expiratory pressure breathing in hospitalized subjects with cystic fibrosis. *Physical Therapy* 2005; 85(12):1278-1289.

Chapter 3

High-Frequency Chest Wall Oscillation Waveforms: Clinical Implications

Kumari Sulochana[1,*], MScRT, FNIV, PhD (Scholar)
Kishore Kumar[2], MScRT, FNIV, PhD (Scholar)
George Savio Chellam[3], MScRT
and Antonio M. Esquinas[4], MD, PhD, FCCP, FNIV

[1]Bharati Hospital and Research Centre, Pune, India
[2]Department of Respiratory Medicine,
Chettinad Academy of Research and Education, Chennai, India
[3]Symbiosis University Hospital and Research Centre, Pune, India
[4]Intensive Care Unit. Hospital Morales Meseguer Murcia, Spain

Abstract

HCWO is a type of airway clearance technique used by physicians, respiratory therapists, physiotherapists, and nurses to enhance the clearance of excess bronchial secretions in patients with chronic obstructive airway disorders. There is no standard term in literature, the terms high-frequency chest wall oscillation (HFCWO) and high-frequency chest wall compression (HFCC) are often used interchangeably. Each high-frequency airway clearance system has unique pressure pulse characteristics (i.e., waveforms and magnitudes) that change with the frequency and pressure settings. Physicians and respiratory therapists recommend therapeutic pressure and frequency settings to meet individual needs. The therapeutic results are also influenced by vest fit (size and snugness), and the frequency, pressure and waveform of the air pulse generated by the system. Different

---

[*] Corresponding Author's Email: sulochana.rt@gmail.com.

In: High-frequency Chest Wall Oscillation Therapy in Critical Ill Patients
Editor: Antonio M. Esquinas
ISBN: 979-8-89530-264-4
© 2025 Nova Science Publishers, Inc.

waveforms (Square, Sine, Triangle) are generated at a specific frequency and pressure setting on the HFCC device. The best frequencies for patient therapy are those that produce the highest airflows and largest volumes. The purpose of this review is to understand the role of HFCWO/HFCC its waveforms in bronchial hygiene therapy and its effectiveness in airway clearance in patients with obstructive airway disorders.

Keywords: high-frequency chest wall oscillation, waveforms, airway clearance device, COPD, cystic fibrosis

Introduction

Chest physiotherapy and airway clearance devices (assisted or unassisted) are important tools in the treatment of obstructive airway disorders such as Cystic Fibrosis, COPD, Bronchiectasis etc. In this chapter, we will only discuss assisted airway clearance devices. There are 3 types of "assisted" high-frequency airway clearance devices: Intrapulmonary percussive ventilation (IPPV), High-frequency chest wall compression (HFCC) devices & High-frequency chest wall oscillation devices (HFCWO) [1].

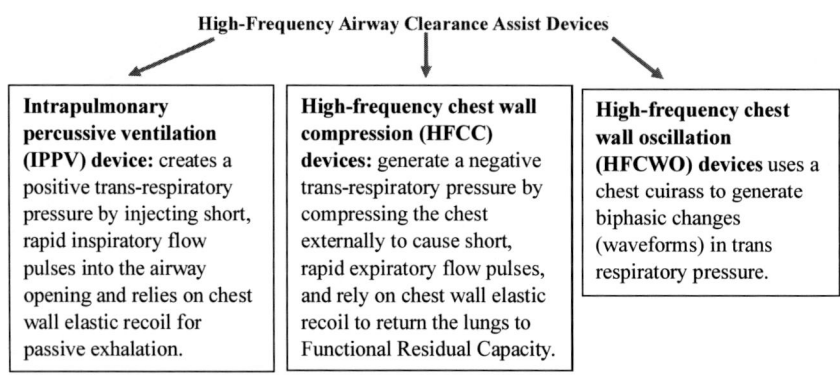

Figure 1. High-Frequency Airway Clearance Assist Devices.

All these high-frequency "assist" airway clearance devices work on the principle of trans-respiratory pressure change which is defined as a change in the pressure difference between the pressure at the airway opening and the pressure on the body surface. In any of these 3 cases (positive or negative pressure pulses or both), the main working principle is to get the air behind the secretions and augment mucus movement toward the larger airway where they can be coughed up and expectorated [1]. Their mechanism of action is shown in Figure 1. As per the literature, there is no standard terminology; the terms high-frequency chest wall oscillation (HFCWO) and high-frequency chest wall compression (HFCC) are often used interchangeably.

HFCWO-HFCC System

HFCWO is achieved with a rigid chest cuirass connected to a compressor that can deliver both positive and negative pressures to the chest wall. High-frequency oscillations are generated using an apparatus known as an oscillating motor. An air compressor and a vest that fits over the torso are used with the motor. The vest contains inflatable bladders connected to the compressor via long, flexible tubing (Figure 2). The compressor pumps bursts of air at varying frequencies (1-20 Hz) and varying pressures into the bladders within the vest. These oscillating motors create individual pressure waveforms that closely mimic manual CPT, the bursts of air entering the vest bladder transmit oscillations or vibrations to the chest wall producing a shearing force on secretions within the airways and increasing airflow into and out of the airways [1, 2]. These varying airflow patterns (inspiratory and expiratory flow ratios) change the physical nature of the mucus, breaking it down and ultimately allowing it to be moved to the central airways where it is coughed out or swallowed. Details in Figure 3.

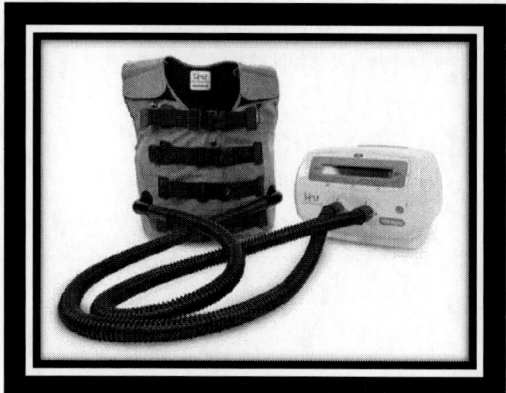

Figure 2. HFCWO system- consists of the Air-Pulse machine (compressor), vest or jacket and tubings (Hillrom™ Vest Airway Clearance System Model 105).

Initially, HFCC was only used for young adults with CF, but now it is also used in those who require long-term airway clearance therapy such as those who have undergone heart/lung transplantation and those with respiratory pump dysfunction secondary to chronic neuromuscular disorders [1]. HFCCs have become ubiquitous enough to constitute a standard of care. Yet, despite many years of research, and clinical evidence of efficacy; their usage in chronic obstructive pulmonary disease patients is still underrated.

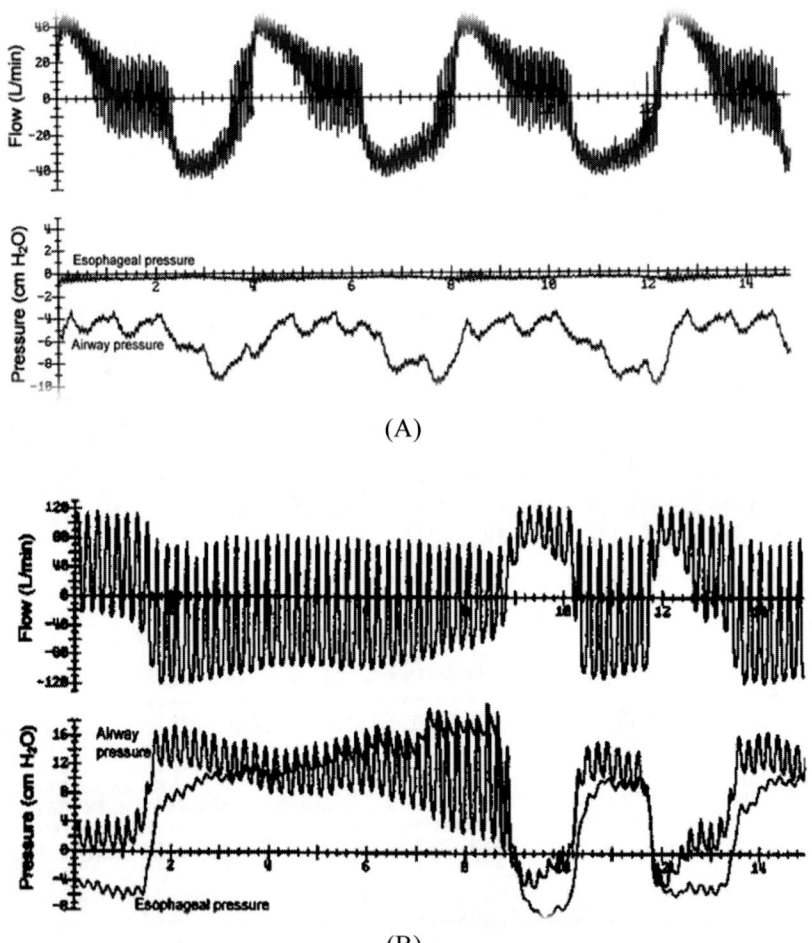

(A)

(B)

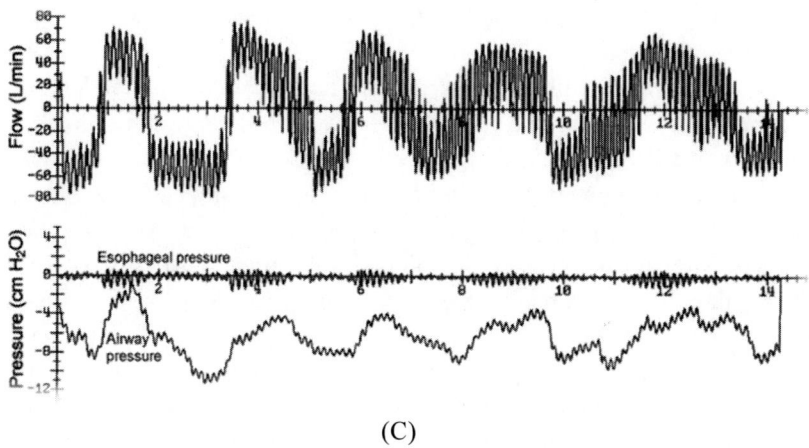

(C)

Figure 3. Shows the Flow, airway pressure, and oesophageal pressure waveforms while breathing through various High-frequency airway clearance devices (A). High-frequency chest wall compresions) (B) Intrapulmonary percusive decive), (C) High-frequency chest wall oscillations).

Basic Waveforms, Frequency and Amplitude of High-Frequency Airway Clearance Device

Although all the high-frequency airway clearance device shares the same fundamental components, but their resulting percussive waveforms are different from each other (Figure 2). Current HFCC machines can be distinguished by their pressure waveforms, which are defined by amplitude and frequency. The frequency is measured in cycles (number of peak waves) per second or Hertz (Hz). At the air pulse generator, each frequency (1-20 Hz) produces a distinct pressure waveform that makes the vest expand and shrink rapidly providing compression to the chest 5-20 times/second [2, 3]. The effectiveness of therapy and patient comfort is dependent on the different frequency and pressure combinations that we use.

HFCWO/HFCC Waveforms

Professor George D. O'clock and colleagues created an HFCC-Lung simulation model to comprehend the energy transfer process and waveform creation by HFCC devices. Details in Figure 4 [4]. For which an HFCC pump–vest and half chest–lung simulation, with 23 lung generations, was developed using inertance, compliance, viscous friction relationships, and Newton's second law. As a result, the simulation showed variations in the structure and intensity of HFCC waveforms in different parts of the pulmonary system [4]. In Figure 5, we show a subject wearing an HFCC vest with hoses attached to the HFCC pump. A pneumotachometer, equipped with a sensing unit to measure airflow and pressure (RespirTech inCourage System-ICS), is placed at the mouth. It is already known that the chest–lung system follows a conventional pressure–airflow–volume relationship to resistance, inertance, and compliance. However, Resonance in human lungs is often described in the range of 4–8 Hz for adults and 10–12 Hz for small infants. Altogether, the resonant frequency for the combination of chest wall, lung tissue, and airway systems has been given as 7–12 Hz for adults. Using an operating frequency of 6 Hz, the effect of intrathoracic resistance was investigated. Figure 4 displays the HFCC-simulated pressure waveforms at different places, including the source (pump), vest, pleural space, lung Generations, and mouth [4]. Here, the pressure waveform is generated at the air pulse generator (P_d), and then this compressive force generated at the inner surface of the vest is transmitted to the chest (P_j), producing oscillatory airflow measurable at the mouth (F_m). These waveforms can be modified by selecting a specific frequency and pressure setting on the HFCC device. Let us understand this with an example; P_d for the 101 and 102 (American Biosystems, Inc., Stillwater, MN)- generates Square Waveform; the 103, 104, 105 (Hill-Rom, St. Paul, MN) and Smart Vest (Electromed, Inc, New Prague, MN)- generates Sine waveforms; and the InCourage System (ICS) (RespirTech, Inc, St. Paul, MN)- generates triangle waveform. In Figure 6 we present a schematic diagram of internal circuits and the pressure waveforms generated by the HFCC system at the (input) pump--vest--chest--pleural space--pulmonary systems and systems interface (mouth). HFCC-induced pressure waveforms at various locations show how the HFCC waveform shape changes as it progresses from the pump to the mouth.

1. The "square" waveform, created in the late 1980s, was the first HFCC waveform [4, 6-7]. The source of the air-pulse generator produced this square waveform. Later, to optimise this technology an air pulse unit (with a square waveform technology) along with active venting capabilities was connected to a vest, and this resulted in a "triangle" waveform [4, 5]. However, the Sine waveform technology was first

presented in 1995; in contrast, triangle waveform systems have been around for ten years and both work in very different ways [3, 5]. An adult HFCC vest's oscillatory recording of a 5-Hz pulse delivered with the sine waveform (diag.1) and triangle waveform (diag.2) differs from one another, as shown in Figure 7. In both cases, the resulting pulse pressure is 11 mm Hg and 23 mm Hg. Clinical evidence from the literature indicates that the waveform's shape influences mucus clearance by HFCC in the following ways: Airflow at the mouth is a commonly used method to assess HFCC effectiveness. Triangle waveforms have been demonstrated to generate less energy directed to the chest and more airflow at the mouth [7, 8, 10]. Theoretically, the HFCC system with the highest efficiency produces the optimum airflow at the mouth using the least amount of energy.

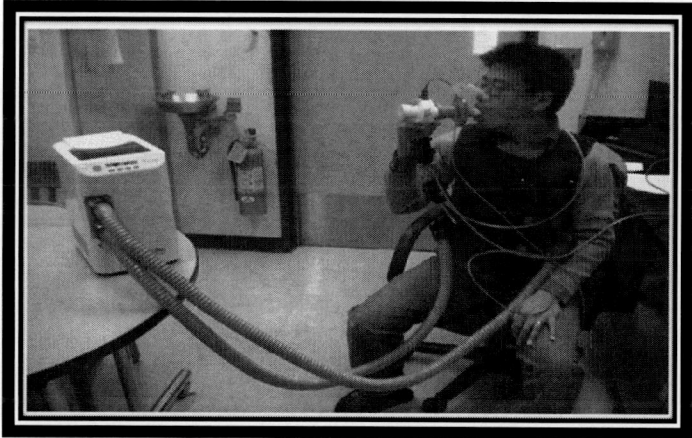

Figure 4. Subject wearing an HFCC vest with hoses connected to the HFCC pump. A pneumotachometer is placed at the mouth with a sensing unit to measure airflow and pressure (RespirTech inCourage System-ICS).

2. The triangle waveform creates peak air pulse pressure for a shorter duration than sine waves [9-10]. This shorter application of peak pressure and lower trough pressure allows the user to take less restricted, deeper breaths, bringing more air into the lungs, which the vest can then force out. This sharper peak produces a rapid "thump" to the chest—an effect similar to manual CPT, but in a manner that is more consistent, repeatable and numerous (typically 6 to 15 cycles

per second). In a typical 30-minute HFCC therapy session with a triangle waveform system, a patient will receive more than 18,000 "thumps."

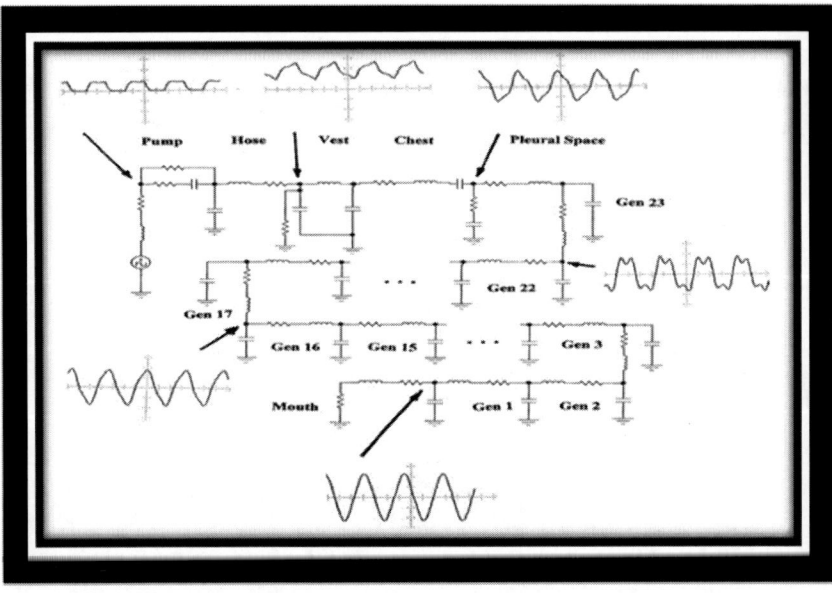

Figure 5. Schematic diagram of internal circuits and the pressure waveforms generated by the HFCC system at the (input) pump--vest--chest--pleural space--pulmonary systems and systems interface (mouth). HFCC-induced pressure waveforms at various locations show how the HFCC waveform shape changes as it progresses from the pump to the mouth.

3. HFCC oscillatory airflow in the lungs is considered a major factor in moving mucus. Triangle waveform is more effective than sine waveform in mucus clearing, delivering a 20% increase in sputum production [9]. This improvement is thought to be due to both the highest airflows and largest air volumes occurring over the same frequency range (5-11 Hz), which may produce greater mucus-shearing force. In contrast, sine waveforms produce the largest volumes at one end of the frequency range (5-11 Hz), and the largest airflows at the other end of the range (15-20 Hz) [8-10].

The best frequencies for patient therapy are those that produce the highest airflows and largest volumes. Another possibility for the difference in mucus-clearing performance is that the triangle waveform has greater pulse pressure because of higher peak and lower trough pressures. The "thump" of a sharp pressure increases, and immediate release creates an airflow bias, which can act to dislodge mucus. A larger airflow bias is created through larger pressure differences, and a larger airflow bias contributes to higher air velocity than occurs with normal breathing.

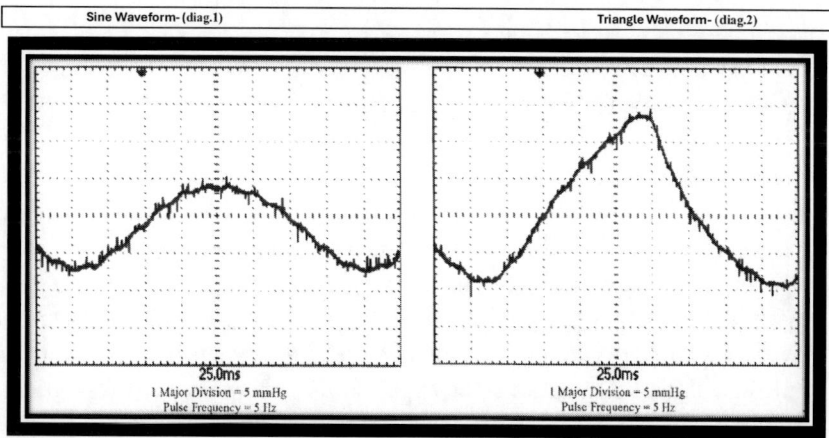

Figure 6. Oscillatory recording of a pulse of 5 Hz delivered with the sine waveform (diag.1) and triangle waveform (diag.2) in an adult HFCC vest. The pulse pressure is 11 mm Hg and 23 mm Hg respectively.

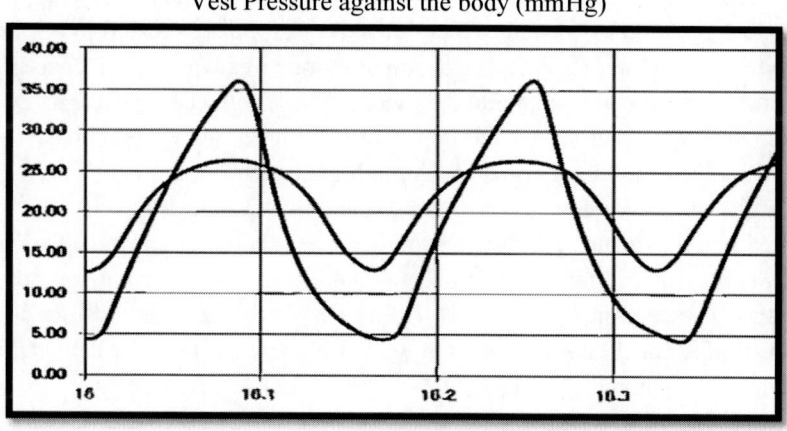

Figure 7. Pressure waveform shape (triangle and sine mmHg) depicted at 6 Hz frequency measured inside the vests.

4. Patients can tolerate the higher peak pressures produced by triangle waveforms because that maximum level of pressure is applied very briefly. Patients perceive sine waveforms at an equivalent peak pressure as uncomfortable (or as one paper put it: "crushing and intolerable") because the maximum pressure occurs for a longer duration with the sine wave's rounded peak [7].

Active Venting for Deeper Inhalations, More Air Movement

When a breath is taken, the chest wall expands. This action pushes the chest against the interior of the pressurized HFCC vest. In an open, triangle-wave producing system, air in the vest is released into the atmosphere both in response to the user's breath and through the cycling of air pulses/spikes produced by the system's patented air chopping system [10]. Sharp peak waveforms are created through "active venting" where air inflow ceases immediately, and the pressure rise experiences a sharp drop off. The triangle waveform's sharper peaks and resulting sudden impact loosen and move mucus through the lungs and airways. Also, the combination of the triangle wave system's lower base pressure and active venting allows the chest to easily expand for deeper, more comfortable breaths during therapy.

In a closed, sine wave-producing system, a mechanical diaphragm squeezes the air back and forth within the system like a bellows mechanism to create surges in airflow rather than the abrupt air pulses created in a triangle wave system. Compressions and decompressions create pressure increases and decrease and produce a natural sine wave. These rounded waveforms do not yield the kind of percussive "thump" that a triangle wave system does.

Sine wave systems also start with a higher base pressure in the vest than triangle waveform devices. A closed, sine wave system vest acts somewhat like a blood pressure cuff around the chest. As the chest expands, the space between the chest and the vest decreases. Because the air cannot escape the system, pressure on the patient is increased, which can result in a feeling of constriction for the user. Details in waveform shape difference depicted at 6 Hz frequency in pressure oscillations measured inside the vests.

Triangle Waveform for Patient Comfort, Therapy Adherence, Secretion Clearance

Though both sine wave and triangle wave devices apply oscillations to the chest wall, there is a difference in how those oscillations are delivered. Patient comfort is a key factor in therapy adherence. In a comparison, vest users reported easier breathing during therapy with a triangle waveform system than with a sine wave system [10]. It stands to reason that the more comfortable the therapy is, the higher the likelihood of adhering to a prescribed regimen. Active venting is designed to enhance patient comfort as well as contribute to triangle waveform development that produces mucus shearing, breakdown and movement. Individual therapy needs to determine the types of interventions best suited for desired outcomes. HFCC should be used for patients with pacemakers and subcutaneous devices.

Conclusion

High-frequency airway clearance devices such as HFCWO/HFCC are beneficial for maintaining a patent airway by effectively clearing out the secretions and improving the pulmonary function of patients with impaired mucociliary clearance. The pressure waveform in the HFCC system is generated at the source air pulse generator and then the compressive force generated at the inner surface of the vest is transmitted to the chest, producing oscillatory airflow measurable at the mouth. Different waveforms (Square, Sine, Triangle) can be generated by selecting a specific frequency and pressure setting on the HFCC device. The best frequencies for patient therapy are those that produce the highest airflows and largest volumes. HFCC efficacy is measured by airflow at the mouth. Triangle waveforms produce more airflow than the sine wave at the mouth with less applied energy to the chest. Active venting in the vest HFCC is designed to generate triangle waveforms which enhance patient comfort (users reported easier breathing during therapy). The triangle waveform creates peak air pulse pressure for a shorter duration than sine waves. This shorter application of peak pressure and lower trough pressure allows the user to take less restricted, deeper breaths, bringing more air into the lungs, which the vest can then force out. HFCC oscillatory airflow in the lungs is considered a major factor in moving mucus. Triangle waveform is more effective than sine waveform in mucus clearing, delivering a 20%

increase in sputum production. This improvement is thought to be due to both the highest airflows and largest air volumes occurring over the same frequency range (5-11 Hz), which may produce greater mucus-shearing force.

Key Messages

1. High-frequency airway clearance is a key technical mechanical approach for airway secretion clearance in a wide spectrum of respiratory disorders. Patients who require mechanical ventilation and secretion clearance can benefit from its use.
2. It is imperative that patients already receiving mechanical ventilation on HFCWO be treated with the proper equipment and settings. Therefore, for the right setup and tools, a fundamental waveform analysis of the HFCWO device and mechanical ventilator is essential.

References

[1] Flume P. A., Robinson K. A., O'Sullivan B. P., Finder J. D., et al. Cystic fibrosis pulmonary guidelines: airway clearance therapies. *Respir Care* 2009;54(4):522-537.

[2] Kempainen R. R., Williams C. B., Hazelwood A., Rubin B. K,. Milla C. E. Comparison of high-frequency chest wall oscillation with differing waveforms for airway clearance in cystic fibrosis. *Chest* 2007;132(4):1227–32.

[3] Lee Y. W., Warwick W. J. The comparison of three high-frequency chest compression devices. *Biomed Instrum Technol* 2008;42:68-75.

[4] O'Clock, G. D., Y. Wan Lee, J. Lee, and W. J. Warwick, "A Simulation Tool to Study High-Frequency Chest Compression Energy Transfer Mechanisms and Waveforms for Pulmonary Disease Applications," in *IEEE Transactions on Biomedical Engineering*, vol. 57, no. 7, pp. 1539-1546, July 2010, doi: 10.1109/TBME.2010.2041453.

[5] Quissesa A., Chris Veronika Gultom E. High-frequency chest wall oscillation: airway clearance management for obstructive pulmonary disease patients. Vol. 9, *Nursing Current* 2021.

[6] Milla C. E., Hansen L. G., Weber A., Warwick W. J. Highfrequency chest compression: effect of a third-generation compression waveform. *Biomed Instrum Technol* 2004;38:322-328.

[7] Sohn, K., W. J. Warwick, Y. W. Lee, J. Lee, and J. Holte, "Investigation of non-Uniform airflow signal oscillation during high-frequency chest compression," *Biomed. Eng. Line*, vol. 4, p. 34, 2005.

[8] Lee, Y. W., J. Lee, and W. J. Warwick, "Waveforms of high-frequency chest compression systems change with jacket, body," *Biomed. Instrum. Technol* 2008. vol. 42, pp. 407–411.

[9] Milla C. E., Hansen L. G., Warwick W. J. Different frequencies should be prescribed for different high-frequency chest compression machines. *Biomed Instrum Technol* 2006;40:319-324.

[10] Tangen, N. Optimization of Secretion Clearance with the HFCC. *Triangle Waveform 2016*, Feb.

Chapter 4

High-Frequency Chest Wall Oscillation: Equipment

Mostafa Elshazly, MD
and Ahmed Tantawy*, MD
Faculty of Medicine, Cairo University, Giza, Egypt

Abstract

High-frequency chest wall oscillation (HFCWO) is a well-established airway clearance approach that has been demonstrated as a therapy to help clear the lungs of secretions in patients with different types of lung disease (cystic fibrosis (CF), bronchiectasis, and COPD) or in certain neurodegenerative disease states in patient populations who are unable to clear secretions from the lungs (ALS, Parkinson's Disease).

Keywords: airway clearance, secretion removal, intrapulmonary percussive ventilation, high-frequency chest wall oscillation

Introduction

While there have long been methods for enhancing the lungs' natural cough clearing and mucociliary processes, several pleasant and efficient methods have emerged in recent years [1]. Most adults and teenagers can apply these

---

* Corresponding Author's Email: ahmedtantawy12@yahoo.com.

In: High-frequency Chest Wall Oscillation Therapy in Critical Ill Patients
Editor: Antonio M. Esquinas
ISBN: 979-8-89530-264-4
© 2025 Nova Science Publishers, Inc.

tactics on their own without assistance. High-frequency airway clearance techniques fall into 2 broad categories: unassisted and assisted.

The energy from passive exhalation is used by unassisted ways to produce vibrations in the chest wall, like the Acapella, the Flutter, the Quake, and the Lung Flute [2].

In assisted techniques, the devices target mucus movement towards the airway opening through a variety of mechanisms, either by increasing trans respiratory pressure associated with flow in the inspiratory direction or by decreasing trans respiratory pressure associated with flow in the expiratory direction. Intrapulmonary percussive devices (IIPV), high-frequency chest wall oscillation (HFCWO), and high-frequency chest wall compression (HFCWC) are examples of active devices [2].

In these aspects, we consider the following basic concepts:

1. Intrapulmonary percussive ventilation (IPV): creates positive changes in trans respiratory difference by injecting short, rapid inspiratory flow pulses into the airway opening and relies on chest wall elastic recoil for passive exhalation.
2. High-frequency chest wall compression (HFCWC): generates negative changes in trans respiratory pressure difference by compressing the chest externally (i.e., body surface pressure goes positive relative to the pressure at the airway opening, which remains at atmospheric pressure) to cause short, rapid expiratory flow pulses, and relies on chest wall elastic recoil to return the lungs to functional residual capacity.
3. High-frequency chest wall oscillation (HFCWO): uses a chest cuirass to generate biphasic changes in trans respiratory pressure difference. In any case (positive or negative pressure pulses or both), the general idea is to augment mucus movement toward the airway opening by a variety of mechanisms.

A well-proven method for clearing secretions from the lungs, high-frequency chest wall oscillation (HFCWO) (Figure 1) has been shown to be effective in treating patients with a variety of lung diseases, including CF, bronchiectasis, and COPD, as well as in certain neurodegenerative disease states where patients are unable to clear secretions from the lungs, such as ALS and Parkinson's disease. High-frequency oscillator for the chest wall (Figure 1).

Table 1. HFCWO device descriptions

Device Name FDA Approval Date	Manufacturer	Features
Frequencer V2 and V2x [5] January 26, 2011 [6]	Dymedso	Portable • Not wearable • 4 sizes of adaptors for patients of different sizes • Generates low frequency sound waves within the range of 20- 65 Hz and offers an adjustable intensity based on the patient's condition
SmartVest SQL System [7] December 19, 2013 [8]	Electromed	• Portable • Wearable • 8 different sizes • 16 pounds • Quiet (60 decibels) • 91% decompression (greater percent decompression than other vests) • Wireless capabilities that can connect usage to personal reports or to healthcare provider records
The Vest Airway Clearance System Model 105 [9] February 21, 2003 [10]	Hill-Rom	Portable • Wearable • 4 styles of garment for different body types (full garment, wrap garment, chest garment, C3 garment) • 17 pounds • Multiple programing options, including several languages • Can program a reminder to cough • Vest covers are washable and dryable • Offers at-home training • Wireless capabilities that can connect usage to personal reports or to healthcare provider records
Respin [11] July 13, 2012 [12]	RespInnovation SAS	Portable • Wearable • Vest plus control unit weight 11 kilograms • Several sizes for different sizes • Can target specific chest areas • Programmable with several protocols • Uses an air pressure piston which inflates and completely empties each cycle enabling the patient to breathe, speak and cough without restriction • Does not provide constant background pressure which manufacturer claims makes the therapy easy to tolerate and puts no pressure onto the patient's physiological state
In Courage Vest [13] June 17, 2005 [14]	Philips, via RespirTech	• Portable • Wearable • Available in 7 sizes • Battery-operated • Has eight mechanical oscillating motors that target all 5 lobes of the lungs, front and back, for fully mobile use • Programmable settings •Advertised as the lightest vest option (no weight specified)
AffloVest [15] March 27, 2013 [10]	International Biophysics Corporation	Portable • Wearable • Available in 7 sizes • Battery-operated • Has eight mechanical oscillating motors that target all 5 lobes of the lungs, front and back, for fully mobile use • Programmable settings

Abbreviations. COPD: chronic obstructive pulmonary disorder; FDA: US Food and Drug Administration; HFCWO: high-frequency chest wall oscillation.

With HFCWO, a pulse generator is mechanically connected to an inflatable jacket worn over the torso via hoses, allowing the device to operate at different frequencies (5–25 Hz) (Figure 2). The patient sat up straight in his chair [2]. The vest rapidly inflates and deflates because of air being sent through the hose by the generator. Mucus is helped to ascend into the larger airways by the vibrations, which also aid to detach it from the walls of the airways [3].

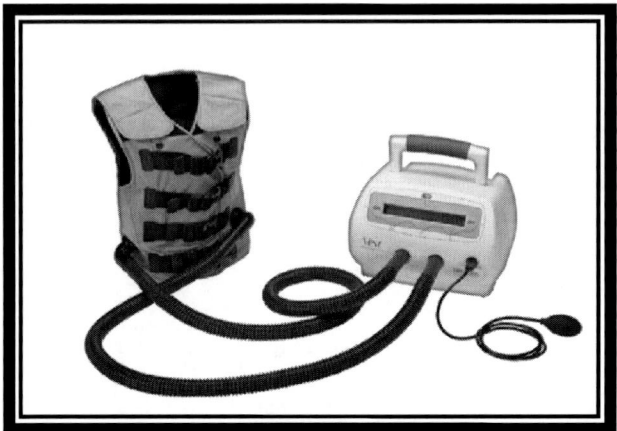

Figure 1. High-frequency chest wall oscillator.

A – Optional remote control port
B – Easy to read display screen
C – Air Hose connection ports
D – Frequency or Hertz (Hz)
E – Pressure
F – Time

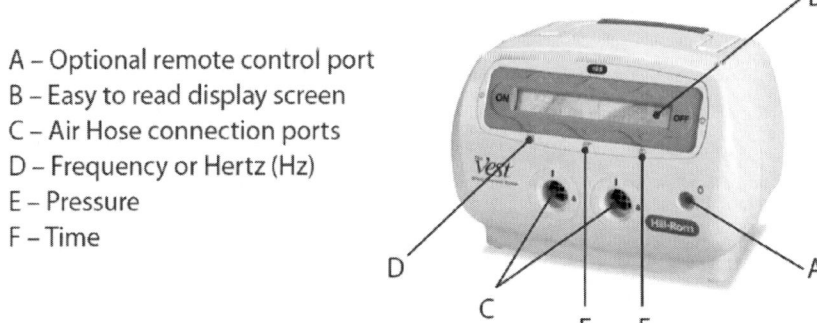

Figure 2. Air pulse generator.

A typical treatment lasts 20–30 min and is interspersed with additional treatments, generally huff coughing and nebulized medications to better expel mucus. Treatments are typically prescribed at least twice daily [4]. Details in Figure 2 and Table 1.

Mechanisms

Many mechanisms have been proposed to explain the effects of assisted airway clearance techniques on mucus transport [4]. The most obvious explanation is that mucus secretion is enhanced by air-liquid shear forces when expiratory flow is higher than inspiratory flow, just as with a normal cough [5, 6]. High-frequency devices simply stack many "mini coughs" into one spontaneous exhalation. High-frequency oscillations may have a mucolytic effect on bronchial secretions [7-10]. Oscillation of the chest might stimulate the vagus nerve through reflex pathways in the airway walls or in the chest wall and may be associated with enhancement of mucociliary beating. To begin your treatment, we may follow these steps summary in Table 2.

There are now one nonwearable HFCWO device and five wearable HFCWO devices that have been approved by the US Food and Drug Administration (FDA) and being manufactured for use in children and adults with cystic fibrosis, bronchiectasis, COPD, or pulmonary complications from neuromuscular disease resulting in chronic lung disease [11-14]. Description of each device and for harms and adverse events in Table 2 and Table 3.

Table 2. Setting for High-frequency chest wall oscillation [9]

1.	With device plugged in, press the Up arrow above normal.
2.	The first number you will see in the upper left-hand corner is the Frequency or Hertz (Hz). Adjust as needed to match your prescription above by using the Up or Down arrows.
3.	The middle number on the screen is the pressure. This should be set based on your garment style. It can also be adjusted by pressing the Up or Down arrows.
4.	The last number on top is the time of your treatment. Adjust as needed to match your prescription above by using the Up and Down arrows.
5.	These settings will be saved as entered for your next treatment.
6.	At this point you are ready to begin. Follow prompts on screen.
7.	Press -ON- to Inflate.
8.	Start Therapy Press- ON.
9.	To pause, press the OFF button or squeeze the remote control once. The unit will stop the pulsations and the garment will deflate. To resume treatment, press the -ON- button or squeeze the Remote Control again.
10.	If it is necessary to end the treatment session before it is complete, press the -OFF- button twice.
11.	When the treatment session is complete, the pulsations will stop, the garment will deflate, and it will read "Session Complete."
12.	Unplug the system from its power source.

Table 3. Adverse events reported in MAUDE by HFCWO device

Device Name FDA Approval Date	Manufacturer	Adverse Event(s)
Frequencer V2 and V2x [5] January 26, 2011 [6]	Dymedso	• No records
SmartVest SQL System [7] December 19, 2013 [8]	Electromed	• No records
The Vest Airway Clearance System Model 105 [9] February 21, 2003 [10]	Hill-Rom	• No records
Respin [11] July 13, 2012 [12]	RespInnovation SAS	• No records
In Courage Vest [13] June 17, 2005 [14]	Philips, via RespirTech	8 reports identified classified under injury event type • Rib bone fractures in 3 different patients • 1 vertebral fracture • 1 electromagnetic interference problem with a pacemaker • 1 hematoma • 1 pneumothorax • 1 pressure problem with co-occurring mastitis
AffloVest [15] March 27, 2013 [10]	International Biophysics Corporation	1 report identified • Fractured ribs

Abbreviations. FDA: US Food and Drug Administration; HFCWO: high-frequency chest wall oscillation; MAUDE: manufacturer and user facility device experience database.

Conclusion

High-frequency chest wall oscillation (HFCWO) is a form of chest physical therapy in which an inflatable vest is attached to a machine that vibrates it at high-frequency. The vest vibrates the chest to loosen and thin mucus that can be cleared by coughing or suctioning [15].

Key Messages

1. High-frequency chest wall oscillation (HFCWO) is an easy-to-use medical device for children and adults who have excess airway mucus and difficulty clearing it effectively.
2. Designed for in-home use, The equipment is quite comfortable, and portable; its features promote user independence and helps simplify treatment routines.

References

[1] Andrews J, Sathe NA, Krishnaswami S, McPheeters ML. Nonpharmacologic airway clearance techniques in hospitalized patients: a systematic review. *Respir Care* 2013;58(12):2160-2186.

[2] Nicolini A, Cardini F, Landucci N, Lanata S, Ferrari-Bravo M, Barlascini C. Effectiveness of treatment with high-frequency chest wall oscillation in patients with bronchiectasis. *BMC Pulm Med* 2013; 13:21.

[3] Lechtzin N, Wolfe LF, Frick KD. The impact of high-frequency chest wall oscillation on healthcare use in patients with neuromuscular diseases. *Ann Am Thorac Soc* 2016;13(6):904-90.

[4] Sawicki GS, Sellers DE, Robinson WM. High treatment burden in adults with cystic fibrosis: challenges to disease self-management. *J Cyst Fibros* 2009;8(2):91-6.

[5] Dymedso. Frequencer. 2021; https://dymedso.com/frequencer/. Accessed April 21, 2021.

[6] US Food and Drug Administration. Dymedso Frequencer V2 and Frequencer V2x airway clearance device. 2011; https://www.accessdata.fda.gov/cdrh_docs/pdf10/K103176.pdf. Accessed April 22, 2021.

[7] Electromed Inc. The smart shoice for HFCWO therapy. 2021;https://smartvest.com/smart-choice-for-hfcwotherapy/?gclid=EAIaIQobChMIz92CqbK7gIV2zizAB01yAGgEAAYASAAEgJoaPD_BwE. Accessed April 21, 2021.

[8] US Food and Drug Administration. Special 510(k) summary. 2013; https://www.accessdata.fda.gov/cdrh_docs/pdf13/K132794.pdf. Accessed April 22, 2021.

[9] Hill-Rom Inc. The Vest airway clearance system, model 105. 2021. Accessed April 21, 2021.

[10] US Food and Drug Administration. 510(k) summary of safety and effectiveness. 2013; https://www.accessdata.fda.gov/cdrh_docs/pdf12/K122480.pdf. Accessed April 22, 2021.

[11] RespInnovation. RespIn 11 bronical clearance system. 2021; http://respin11.com/index.php/respin/respin-11. Accessed April 21, 2021.

[12] US Food and Drug Administration. *Premarket notification* 510(k). 2012; https://www.accessdata.fda.gov/cdrh_docs/pdf12/K121170.pdf. Accessed April 22, 2021.

[13] Philips, RespirTech. InCourage system airway clearance device. 2021; https://www.usa.philips.com/healthcare/product/HC500055/incourage system-airway-clearance-device. Accessed April 22, 2021.

[14] US Food and Drug Administration. 510(k) summary of safety and effectiveness. 2005; https://www.accessdata.fda.gov/cdrh_docs/pdf5/K051383.pdf. Accessed April 22, 2021.

[15] International Biophysics Corportation. AffloVest mobile mechanial HFCWO vest therapy. 2020; https://www.afflovest.com/. Accessed Aprik 22, 2021.

Chapter 5

High-Frequency Chest Wall Oscillation: Setting Pressure and Frequency

Mohamad F. El-Khatib*, PhD, MB, RRT
Department of Anesthesiology and Pain Medicine, American University of Beirut, School of Medicine and Medical Center, Beirut, Lebanon

Abstract

High-frequency chest wall oscillation (HFCWO) consists of medical equipment that functions as a pressure generator and an inflatable vest wrapped around the patient's chest. The equipment mechanically performs automated chest physical therapy by vibrating with a certain pressure at a high-frequency. The vest vibrates the chest to loosen and thin mucus. The most important components of HFCWO are how to set both pressure and frequency. The setting of oscillating pressure and frequency depends greatly on the medical equipment used, on the patients' population and characteristics, as well as on the disease entity and severity.

Keywords: oscillating pressure, high-frequency chest wall oscillation, mucus secretion, chest physical therapy

Introduction

High-frequency chest wall oscillation (HFCWO) therapy is an automated form of chest physical therapy intended to help in mobilizing and clearing mucus

---

* Corresponding Author's Email:mk05@aub.edu.lb.

In: High-frequency Chest Wall Oscillation Therapy in Critical Ill Patients
Editor: Antonio M. Esquinas
ISBN: 979-8-89530-264-4
© 2025 Nova Science Publishers, Inc.

and secretions from the airways [1]. HFCWO is commonly prescribed as an airway clearance technique in patients whose ability to expectorate sputum is compromised. The therapy is provided by using a special device that serves as an "air pulse generator" and a patient's garment which is usually an inflatable vest [2]. The device and the vest are connected via a hose. HFCWO can be used in both spontaneously breathing and mechanically ventilated patients as well as in adults and children. Originally used for young adults with cystic fibrosis, HFCWO is now also used in other patients with long-term need for airway clearance such as those who have undergone heart/lung transplantation and those with respiratory pump dysfunction secondary to chronic neuromuscular disorders [3, 4].

In its basic setup, HFCWO consists of an air compressor that delivers oscillating positive and negative pressures (i.e., pressure pulses) to the chest wall at very high frequencies (expressed in Hertz (Hz) and 1 Hz is 60 cycles/minute) to help loosen the mucus and secretions. This rapid inflation and deflation create pressure on the chest similar to clapping. The vibrations not only separate mucus and secretions from the airway walls, but they also help in moving them up into the large airways. Although several variables can be controlled during HFCWO such as the duration of the therapy, the two most important parameters remain the pressure (either in $cmH2O$ or as an arbitrary scale) generated and applied to the vest as well as the frequency of the oscillations expressed in Hz. In this chapter, the focus is on how to set the pressure and frequency during HFCWO therapy.

The specific pressure and frequency settings during HFCWO therapy may vary depending on the patient's needs and the device being used. For proper guidance, it is always advisable to follow the specific instructions provided by the manufacturer and in close coordination with the healthcare care provider. However, some general guidelines for setting the pressure and frequency can be initially applied and followed.

Setting Up the Pressure (P)

The pressure, expressed in $cmH2O$ or as an arbitrary scale, refers to the amplitude or force of the oscillations applied to the chest wall. The appropriate level of pressure applied depends on the individual's tolerance and the severity of the condition. The pressure is often adjustable and can be increased or decreased as needed. It is usually recommended to start with a lower pressure setting and gradually increase it to a patient's comfortable level. Too much pressure can cause discomfort and pain, or intervene with mechanical ventilation, while too little pressure may be ineffective in mobilizing the mucus and secretions. In mechanically ventilated patients secondary to pneumonic respiratory failure, it is advisable to use the lowest pressure settings for HFCWO therapy [3], to minimize the risk of false- or auto-triggering of the mechanical ventilator that can occur when high oscillation pressures are used [4]. In a mix of ICU patients (mechanical ventilation, pneumonia, and chest wall injury), the use of HFCWO at the lowest level of pressure was associated with better comfort, produced an improvement in lung condition, and reduced the number of days to use the ventilator on patients compared to manual percussion of chest physiotherapy [5].

At oscillation pressures as low as 2-5 cmH2O, HFCWO produced an improvement in several lung function parameters compared to traditional chest physiotherapy in patients with bronchiectasis [6]. When the same level of oscillation pressures (2-5 cmH2O) was applied to patients with severe COPD, significant improvements in the tests of dyspnea and daily life activity evaluations compared to standard physiotherapy, as well as in pulmonary function tests (e.g., forced vital capacity, forced expiratory volume in 1 second, forced expiratory volume in 1 second/forced vital capacity%, total lung capacity, residual volume, carbon monoxide diffusing lung capacity, maximal inspiratory pressure, maximal expiratory pressure) and arterial blood gas values were observed [7]. HFCWO has been attempted on patients with COVID-19 using high oscillating pressures (75% of Pmax) and low frequencies. When compared with standard physiotherapy technique, HFCWO at high oscillating pressures improved the forced expiratory volume in 1 second, forced vital capacity, peak expiratory flow rates as well as oxygen saturation [8]. HFCWO was well tolerated by COVID-19 patients and resulted in fewer number of patients requiring non-invasive mechanical ventilation [8]. In adult patients with acute exacerbation of their CF, HFCWO at mid-pressure ranges (50% of Pmax) improved ventilation distribution, gas mixing, and lung function [9]. Similar findings were reported when the pressure was set as per the patient's comfort and tolerance in patients with acute exacerbation of CF [10].

Setting Up the Frequency (F)

The frequency refers to the number of oscillations per minute. It is expressed in hertz (Hz) and most of the available devices allow a frequency range between 1 and 20 Hz (i.e., 60 to 1,200 oscillations per minute). Lower frequencies are usually used in children or individuals with more delicate chest walls while higher frequencies are used with older children and adults. The addition of HFCWO therapy at frequencies in the range of 10-15 Hz to standard medical treatment of adult patients with cystic fibrosis (CF) decreases airway obstruction and benefits CF patients during acute respiratory exacerbation [9]. Frequencies in the range of 10-12 Hz have been used successfully in mechanically ventilated patients because of respiratory failure due to pneumonia [3]. In a mixed ICU population with different etiology, frequencies in the range of 10-15 Hz were well tolerated during HFCWO [5]. Higher frequencies in the range of 13-15 Hz can be applied in adult patients with bronchiectasis. At such high frequencies, the HFCWO technique provided an improvement both in pulmonary function and quality of life-related parameters in patients with chronic hypersecretive disease [6]. HFCWO at high frequencies of 13-15 can improve daily life activities and lung function in patients with severe COPD [7]. At a frequency of 8 Hz, HFCWO resulted in significant improvements in oxygenation by providing significant improvements in the pulmonary function of COVID-19 patients [8]. During the acute stage of exacerbation of CF, HFCWO at frequencies in the 10-15 Hz range resulted in improvements in FVC and FEV1. Also, ventilation distribution and gas mixing were improved with HFCWO therapy [9] (Table 1).

Table 1. General guideline for setting pressure and frequency during high-frequency chest wall oscillation

Category	Pressure	Frequency
Acute exacerbation of CF	50% of maximum level	10-15 Hz
Adult Cystic Fibrosis	6-9 cmH2O	9-12 Hz
Bronchiectasis	2-5 cmH2O	13-15 Hz
COPD	2-5 cmH2O	13-15 Hz
COVID-19	75% of maximum Pressure	8 Hz
ICU patients	Least amount of comfortable pressure	10-15 Hz
Mechanically Ventilated Patients	10-20% of maximum Pressure	10-12 Hz

Conclusion

High-frequency chest wall oscillation (HFCWO) is an airway clearance technique in which external chest wall oscillations with variable intensities and frequencies are applied to the chest using an inflatable vest that wraps around the chest. The objective of the therapy is to help in loosening and thinning mucus and secretions and separate them from the airways. The success of HFCWO therapy depends largely on the implementation of evidence-based protocols in which the application of appropriate levels of pressure and frequencies is vital.

Key Messages

1. High-frequency chest wall oscillation (HFCWO) is an efficient form of chest physical therapy intended to help in mobilizing and clearing mucus and secretions from the airways in patients with compromised mechanisms for clearing secretions from their airways
2. Setting and adjustment of the oscillating pressure and frequency are the cornerstone for efficient HFCWO therapy
3. The appropriate setting of the oscillating pressure depends on the patient's characteristics, the equipment used to provide the therapy, as well as the disease entity.

References

[1] Warnock L, Gates A. Airway clearance techniques compared to no airway clearance techniques for cystic fibrosis. *Cochrane Database Syst Rev* 2023.12;4(4):CD001401.

[2] Nicolini A, Grecchi B, Banfi P. Effectiveness of two high-frequency chest wall oscillation techniques in patients with bronchiectasis: a randomized controlled preliminary study. *Panminerva Med* 2022;64(2):235-243.

[3] Chuang ML, Chou YL, Lee CY, Huang SF. Instantaneous responses to high-frequency chest wall oscillation in patients with acute pneumonic respiratory failure receiving mechanical ventilation A randomized controlled study. *Medicine* 2017, 96:9 (e5912).

[4] Chatburn RL. High-frequency assisted airway clearance. *Respir Care* 2007;52:1224–35.

[5] Lin YP, Tung HH, Wang TJ. Comparative Study of High-frequency Chest Wall Oscillation and Traditional Chest Physical Therapy in Intensive Care Unit Patients. *J Comp Nurs Res Care* 2017, 2:115-118.

[6] Nicolini A, Cardini F, Landucci N, Lanata S, Ferrari-Bravo M, and Barlascini C. Effectiveness of treatment with high-frequency chest wall oscillation in patients with bronchiectasis. *BMC Pulmonary Medicine* 2013, 13:21-28.

[7] Nicolini A, Grecchi B, Ferrari-Bravo M, Barlascini C. Safety and effectiveness of the high-frequency chest wall oscillation vs intrapulmonary percussive ventilation in patients with severe COPD. *International Journal of COPD* 2018:13 617–625.

[8] Çelik M, Yayık AM, Kerget B, Kerget F, Doymuş Ö, Aksakal A, Özmen S, Aslan MH, Uzun Y. High-Frequency Chest Wall Oscillation in Patients with COVID-19: A Pilot Feasibility Study. *Eurasian J Med* 2022 Jun; 54(2): 150–156.

[9] Darbee JC, Kanga JF, Ohtake PJ. Physiologic Evidence for High-Frequency Chest Wall Oscillation and Positive Expiratory Pressure Breathing in Hospitalized Subjects with Cystic Fibrosis. *Physical Therapy* 2005, Volume 85, Issue 12, 1 December 1278–1289.

[10] Osman LP, Roughton M, Hodson ME, Pryor JA. Short-term comparative study of high-frequency chest wall oscillation and European airway clearance techniques in patients with cystic fibrosis. *Thorax* 2010;65:196e200.

Chapter 6

High-Frequency Chest Wall Oscillation: Clinical Monitoring

**Mostafa Elshazly*, MD
and Mohamed Kamal Hasswa, MD**
Faculty of Medicine, Cairo University, Giza, Egypt

Abstract

Mucus secretion in the lungs is a natural process that protects the airways from inhaled insoluble particle accumulation by capture and removal via the mucociliary escalator. Many pathological conditions may result in thickening of the mucus layer and may be associated with high viscosity (as in Cystic fibrosis), leading to airway obstruction and impairing the delivery of inhaled medications to obstructed regions of the lungs, resulting in poorly controlled disease with associated increased morbidity and mortality. High-frequency chest wall oscillation (HFCWO) is a form of chest physical therapy in which an inflatable vest is attached to a machine that vibrates it at high-frequency. The vest vibrates the chest to loosen and thin the mucus. The loosened secretions may require another intervention to be cleared from the airways.

Keywords: high-frequency chest wall oscillation, airway mucus clearance, non-cystic fibrosis bronchiectasis, neuromuscular disorders

---

* Corresponding Author's Email: melshazly@kasralainy.edu.eg.

In: High-frequency Chest Wall Oscillation Therapy in Critical Ill Patients
Editor: Antonio M. Esquinas
ISBN: 979-8-89530-264-4
© 2025 Nova Science Publishers, Inc.

Introduction

High-frequency chest wall oscillation (HFCWO) creates high velocity, low amplitude oscillatory airflows when applied through a pneumatic vest worn over the thorax and is used for airway mucus clearance in patients with cystic fibrosis, bronchiectasis, and neuromuscular disorders [1].

Studies in patients with cystic fibrosis suggest that HFCWO applied via a pneumatic vest is as effective as other modes of airway mucus clearance, including hand-held devices (e.g., flutter devices) and conventional chest physiotherapy [2].

The proposed mechanism of action of HFCWO is enhancement of mucus transport in three essential ways: by altering the rheological properties of mucus, by creating a cough-like expiratory airflow bias that shears mucus from the airway walls, and by enhancing ciliary beat frequency, all of which help move mucus toward central airways [3] (Table 1).

Table 1. Summary of diagnosis and measurements for HFCWO

Diagnosis and background history:
• Complications
• Medications used
• IV antibiotic therapy with dosage, frequency, and duration
• Recent hospitalizations
• School, work, and extracurricular activity absences due to diagnosis-related complications
HFCWO assessment:
Short-term measures
• Observation of respiratory pattern & rate
• Auscultation
• Oxygen saturations
• Cough
• Peak cough flow
• Sputum
• Oxygen requirement
• Number of suctions / catheters used
Long-Term measures
• Lung function test
• Chest x-ray
• Length of treatment
• Exercise tolerance
• Microbiology
• Number of hospital admissions
• Number of respiratory infections
• Number of courses of antibiotics for respiratory infection
• Burden of care
• Number of carers required to perform treatment

In patients with NCFB, the initiation of HFCWO was associated with reductions in patient-reported exacerbation rates, hospitalizations, antibiotic use, and improvements in respiratory symptoms and quality of life. Importantly these benefits were also observed in the frequent exacerbator subgroup. Moreover, the improvements in hospitalizations rates, consistent with self-reported quality of life measures, suggest that patient health improvement is sustained for at least a year after initiating therapy [4].

In a single-center, investigator initiated, prospective study of 22 subjects, assessed the clinical feasibility of HFCWC therapy in neurologically impaired children with respiratory symptoms. The threshold of adherence to the therapy was 70%. The number of pulmonary exacerbations that required hospitalization was recorded, noting 45% of the subjects required hospital admissions before initiation of HFCWC therapy. This rate decreased to 36% after the first year and to 13% after the second year with this therapy. There was a statistically significant reduction of the number of hospital days at follow-up compared to pre-treatment. The authors concluded that regular HFCWC therapy may reduce the number of hospitalizations in neurologically impaired children [5].

Nicolini and colleagues' 2013 RCT, identified in the systematic review, reported a statistically significant decrease in breathlessness, cough and sputum on the Breathlessness, Cough, and Sputum Scale (BCSS) in the group treated with HFCWO devices compared to a control group that received chest physiotherapy (mean difference, -5.8; 95% CI, -7.21 to -4.39; N = 20; P < .05) [6].

In chronic obstructive pulmonary diseases HFCWO produces improvements in gas mixing and homogenization of alveolar ventilation for previously closed or under ventilated lung units [7]. HFCWO has been shown to decrease functional residual capacity (FRC) in subjects with obstructive lung disease, this could explain the improvement of FVC we have observed [7].

Huang et al. aiming to evaluate the efficacy of high-frequency chest wall oscillation for sputum expectoration and hospital length of stay in patients with acute exacerbations of chronic obstructive pulmonary diseases did a systemic review and meta-analysis of 13 randomized controlled trials (included 756 patients) [8]. They found that compared to other airway clearance techniques, HFCWO significantly increased expectorated sputum volume by 6.18 mL (95% CI: 1.71 to 10.64; $I2 = 87\%$), shortened hospital stay by 4.37 days (95% CI: −7.70 to −1.05; $I2 = 84\%$). However, FEV1 (%), PaO2, and PaCO2 did not improve significantly. They concluded that AECOPD patients may benefit from HFCWO therapy. HFCWO enables AECOPD patients to excrete more sputum and shorten their hospital stays. However, due to heterogeneity among the included research, these results should be interpreted with caution

Çelik et al. evaluated the efficacy of high-frequency chest wall oscillation on100 patients with coronavirus disease 2019 pneumonia [9]. High-frequency chest wall oscillation treatment was applied twice a day for 20 minutes for 5 days. No additional interventions were made to the control group. Pulmonary function tests and oxygenation were evaluated on the first and fifth days. Patients' high-flow oxygen, non-invasive mechanical ventilation, and invasive mechanical ventilation needs were evaluated and recorded. They found that compared with the control group, the forced expiratory volume in first second (FEV_1), forced vital capacity (FVC), and peak expiratory flow rates (PEFR) were statistically higher in the rehabilitation group on the fifth day ($p < .05$). On evaluating the oxygenation status of patients, the fifth day to first-day oxygen saturation difference was significantly higher in rehabilitation group than in control group ($p < .05$). Furthermore, the number of patients who needed non-invasive mechanical ventilation was lower in the rehabilitation group ($p < .05$). They concluded that pulmonary rehabilitation applied with the high-frequency chest wall oscillation device in patients with coronavirus disease 2019 in the early period contributed to the improvement of oxygenation by providing significant improvement as observed in the pulmonary function tests of the patients.

Huang et al. studied the effectiveness, safety, and tolerance/comfort of high-frequency chest wall oscillation after extubation in patients with prolonged mechanical ventilation (PMV). Their study was parallel designed, randomized controlled trial enrolled subjects with both intra-tracheal intubation and mechanical ventilator support continuously for at least 21 days [10]. Upon extubation, the participants were randomly assigned to either receive HFCWO for 5 days or not. The effectiveness [based on weaning success rates, daily clearance volume of sputum, serial changes in sputum coloration and chest X-ray (CXR) improvement rates], safety (by physiologic parameters) and tolerance/comfort [using the Modified Borg Scale (MBS) and Hamilton Anxiety Scale (HAS)] of HFCWO were investigated [10].

They found that in 43 PMV subjects, including 23 in the HFCWO group and 20 in the non-HFCWO group. The weaning success rates were 82.6% (19/23) and 85% (17/20) in the HFCWO and non-HFCWO groups, respectively ($P = 1.000$). The HFCWO group had persistently greater numbers of daily sputum suctions and higher CXR improvement rates compared with the non-HFCWO group. There was significant sputum coloration lightening in the HFCWO group only. There was no significant difference in the MBS and HAS between the two groups and between pre- and post-HFCWO physiologic parameters. They concluded that in PMV patients, HFCWO were safe, comfortable, and effective in facilitating airway hygiene after removal of endotracheal tubes but had no positive impact on weaning success. Chuang et al. investigate the effect of HFCWO on pneumonic subjects with acute respiratory failure receiving mechanical ventilation by evaluating immediate cardiopulmonary changes and changes in the initial ventilator settings caused by oscillation [11]. Their study included 73 patients (52 men) aged 71.5 ± 13.4 years who were intubated with mechanical ventilation for pneumonic respiratory failure and randomly classified into 2 groups (HFCWO group, n = 36; and control group who received conventional chest physical therapy (CCPT, n = 37). HFCWO was applied with a fixed protocol, whereas CCPT was conducted using standard protocols. Both groups received sputum suction after the procedure. Changes in ventilator settings and the subjects' responses were measured at preset intervals and compared within groups and between groups. They found that Oscillation did not affect the ventilator settings (all $P > 0.05$). The mean airway pressure, breathing frequency, and rapid shallow breathing index increased, and the tidal volume and SpO2 decreased (all $P < 0.05$). After sputum suction, the peak airway pressure (Ppeak) and minute ventilation decreased (all $P < 0.05$). The HFCWO group had a lower tidal volume and SpO2 at the end of oscillation, and lower Ppeak and tidal volume after sputum suction than the CCPT group. They concluded that HFCWO affects breathing pattern and SpO2 but not ventilator settings, whereas CCPT maintains a steadier condition. After sputum suction, HFCWO slightly improved Ppeak compared to CCPT, suggesting that the study extends the indications of HFCWO for these patients in intensive care unit. In the previously published studies, HFCWO showed the following findings (Table 2).

Table 2. Effects HFCWO

1. Improvement of wet weight sputum or greater sputum expectoration [12].
2. Reduction of dyspnoea (Borg score) [13].
3. Improvement in ventilation distribution and gas mixing [14].
4. Improvement of healthy scores (CAT and BCSS) and quality of life (St Georges Respiratory Questionnaire) [6].
5. Improvement of respiratory function parameters (FVC, and FEV1) and changes in sputum cell counts [6].

Table 3. Contraindications for HFCWO

Absolute contraindications
Unstable head or neck injury
Active haemorrhage with hemodynamic instability
Relative contraindications
Lung contusion.
Osteomyelitis of the ribs.
Rib fracture (Osteoporosis- Coagulopathy-Presence of chest wall pain)

One study demonstrated significant desaturation using HFCWO compared to PEP in patients with moderate to severe disease and recommended oxygen saturation monitoring if used in this patient group [12]. Regarding contraindications in Table 3 we present a summary of contraindications absolute and relative [15].

Conclusion

High-frequency chest wall oscillation is currently being utilized in many acute and chronic respiratory conditions. It is widely prescribed and utilized in conditions such as Cystic Fibrosis, non-Cystic fibrosis Bronchiectasis, COPD and in neuromuscular diseases. HFCWO is a safe and comfortable treatment that can significantly increase both the daily clearance volume of sputum and CXR improvement rates together with lightening sputum coloration within a short period after onset of treatment.

Key Messages

1. HFCWO is a safe and comfortable treatment that can significantly increase both the daily clearance volume of sputum.
2. In mechanically ventilated patients HFCWO did not affect the ventilator settings but did significantly change breathing pattern and increase mean airway pressure, and diastolic blood pressure and modestly decreased SpO2. However, with subsequent sputum suction, HFCWO significantly lowered Ppeak and tended to lower the heart rate as compared to CCPT, suggesting that the study extends the

indications of HFCWO for patients with acute pneumonic respiratory failure in ICU.

References

[1] Arens R, Gozal D, Omlin K, Vega J, Boyd K, Keens T, Woo M: Comparison of high-frequency chest compression and conventional chest physiotherapy in hospitalized patients with cystic fibrosis. *Am J Respir Crit Care Med* 1994, 150:1154-1157.
[2] Morrison L, Agnew J: Oscillation devices for airway clearance in people with cystic fibrosis. *Cochran Database of Systemic Reviews* 2009 2010, CD006842.
[3] Hansen LG, Warwick WJ, Hansen KL. Mucus transport mechanisms in relation to the effect of high-frequency chest compression (HFCC) on mucus clearance. *Pediatr Pulmonol* 1994; 17: 113–118.
[4] Barto TL, Maselli DJ, Daignault S, et al. Real-life experience with high-frequency chest wall oscillation vest therapy in adults with non-cystic fibrosis bronchiectasis. *Therapeutic Advances in Respiratory Disease* 2020; 14.
[5] Fitzgerald K, Dugre J, Pagala S, et al. High-frequency chest wall compression therapy in neurologically impaired children. *Respir Care* 2014 Jan;59(1):107-12.
[6] Nicolini A, Cardini F, Landucci N, Lanata S, Ferrari-Bravo M, Barlascini C. Effectiveness of treatment with high-frequency chest wall oscillation in patients with bronchiectasis. *BMC Pulm Med* 2013; 13:21.
[7] Braveman J, Nozzarella M: High-frequency chest compression advanced therapy for obstructive lung disease. *Resp Therapy* 2007, 2:48–5.1.
[8] Hsiao-Ping Huang, Kee-Hsin Chen, Chen-Liang Tsai, Wen-Pei Chang, Sherry Yueh-Hsia Chiu, Shin-Rou Lin, Yu-Huei Lin: Effects of High-Frequency Chest Wall Oscillation on Acute Exacerbation of Chronic Obstructive Pulmonary Disease: A Systematic Review and Meta-Analysis of Randomized Controlled Trials. *International Journal of Chronic Obstructive Pulmonary Disease* 2022:17 2857–2869.
[9] Mine Çelik, Ahmet Murat Yayık, Buğra Kerget, Ferhan Kerget, Ömer Doymuş, Alperen Aksakal, Sevilay Özmen, Mehtap Hülya Aslan, Yakup Uzun. High-Frequency Chest Wall Oscillation in Patients with COVID-19: A Pilot Feasibility Study. *Eurasian J Med* 2022;54(2):150-156.
[10] Huang W-C, Wu P-C, Chen C-J, Cheng Y-H, Shih S-J, Chen H-C and Wu C-L. High-frequency chest wall oscillation in prolonged mechanical ventilation patients: a randomized controlled trial. *Clin Respir J* 2016; 10: 272– 281.
[11] Ming-Lung Chuang, Yi-Ling Chou, RN, Chai-Yuan Lee, Shih-Feng Huang. Instantaneous responses to high-frequency chest wall oscillation in patients with acute pneumonic respiratory failure receiving mechanical ventilation A randomized controlled study. *Medicine* 2017, 96:9(e5912).
[12] Piquet J, Brochard L, Isabey D, et al. High-frequency chest wall oscillation in patients with chronic air-flow obstruction. *Am Rev Respir Dis* 1987; 136:1355-1359.

[13] Fainardi V, Longo F, Faverzani S, Tripodi MC, Chetta A, Pisi G. Short-term effects of high-frequency chest compression and positive expiratory pressure in patients with cystic fibrosis. *J Clin Med Res* 2011;3(6):279–284.

[14] Darbee JC, Kanga JF, Ohtake PJ. Physiologic evidence for high-frequency chest wall oscillation and positive expiratory pressure breathing in hospitalized subjects with cystic fibrosis. *Phys Ther* 2005; 85:1278–1289.

[15] Strickland SL, Rubin BK, Drescher GS, et al. AARC clinical practice guideline: effectiveness of nonpharmacologic airway clearance therapies in hospitalized patients. *Respir Care* 2013;58(12):2187-2193.

Chapter 7

How to Evaluate High-Frequency Chest Wall Oscillation in Mechanical Ventilation

Cátia Pimentel[*], MD

Department of Pulmonology, Centro Hospitalar de Leiria, Portugal

Abstract

Mechanical ventilation has the potential to improve patients' outcomes especially in acute and chronic respiratory failure. Nevertheless, it has some well-known associated complications, such as impairing the maintenance of airway hygiene. Mucus accumulation is one of the problems seen in those patients, and high-frequency assisted airway clearance systems have the potential to dislocate mucus from the bronchial tree and help to mobilize these secretions. When evaluating the possibility to use the two technologies at the same time, in the same patient, there are concerns about how these high-frequency systems may interfere with the ventilator setting and compromise the patients' ventilation. There have been studies that have shown that ventilator mode, settings of the high-frequency assisted airway clearance systems (as oscillation frequency and pressure setting) interfered with the ventilator respiratory frequency, inspiratory-expiratory flows, and flow bias. Nevertheless, some researchers found that the use of this system in these patients is safe. In prolonged mechanical ventilation patients, these systems appear to be safe, comfortable and effective in facilitating airway hygiene after removal of endotracheal tubes, but their role on weaning success is less clear. In this chapter, all these topics will be discussed, presenting the available and most recent data at the time.

---

[*] Corresponding Author's Email: catia.sa.pimentel@hotmail.com.

In: High-frequency Chest Wall Oscillation Therapy in Critical Ill Patients
Editor: Antonio M. Esquinas
ISBN: 979-8-89530-264-4
© 2025 Nova Science Publishers, Inc.

Keywords: HFCWO, chest physiotherapy, sputum clearance, mechanical ventilator, interactions

Introduction

Mechanical ventilation can be a life-support intervention for patients with respiratory failure. However, it does pose certain risks such as atelectasis and ventilator-associated pneumonia [1]. A common challenge seen in patients with respiratory failure with endotracheal intubation, mechanical ventilation, and sedation is excessive sputum production. The invasive nature of ventilation amplifies the risk of sputum retention due to compromised mucociliary clearance resulting from the presence of the endotracheal tube itself and the effects of the sedative drugs. These patients may therefore have worse bronchial hygiene and ventilation-perfusion mismatches due to lung atelectasis or collapse. Excessive bronchial secretions have been associated with extubation failure, highlighting the need for timely intervention [1].

The maintenance of airway hygiene also becomes compromised in critically ill patients due to impairment of the cough reflex and ineffective mucociliary clearance secondary to sedation, inadequate humidification, elevated concentrations of inspired oxygen, heightened pressure in the endotracheal tube cuff, and inflammation and damage to the tracheal mucosa. Implementing airway clearance strategies, including manual hyperinflation, thorough preoxygenation, and appropriate suctioning techniques, can help mitigate the negative impacts associated with tracheal suctioning. Mucociliary dysfunction is a prevalent issue in both acutely and chronically mechanically ventilated patients, stemming from various factors, which are a direct consequence of mechanical ventilation. Additionally, there are indirect effects arising from comorbid critical illnesses, such as inflammation, immobility, and atelectasis [2].

Anesthetic medications, particularly dexmedetomidine and ketamine, have demonstrated a direct reduction in mucociliary clearance in in vitro models. Additionally, a high fraction of inspired oxygen (FiO2) is known to decrease tracheal mucus velocity, likely attributed to compromised ciliary function. The presence of endotracheal tube cuffs can cause direct epithelial damage, further contributing to impaired ciliary function and reduced tracheal mucus velocity. Among these patients, recurrent pulmonary infections may act as a predisposing factor, exacerbating mucociliary dysfunction. The mechanical obstruction of glottic closure by the endotracheal tube results in impaired cough, and this even more impairment relative immobility and muscle weakness, ultimately leading to increased atelectasis and retention of secretions in these patients [2].

Ventilation and airway hygiene are fundamental in respiratory care for mechanically ventilated patients. This involves optimizing ventilation, ensuring effective airway clearance, preventing pulmonary complications, and speeding up weaning from mechanical ventilation. While pneumonia is not a current indication for chest physical therapy, it's known that acute pneumonic patients with respiratory failure on mechanical ventilation face a potential risk of developing atelectasis or lobar collapse, which could warrant consideration for appropriate interventions [1].

Respiratory physiotherapy aimed at increasing tidal volume may potentially enhance secretion clearance and lung compliance in adults with pneumonia who are under invasive ventilation. However, its effects on various outcomes like mortality, length of stay, and other patient-centered measures remain uncertain. Further research and comprehensive studies are needed to clarify and provide a more detailed understanding of the impact of this intervention.

The mucus clearance modalities for mechanically ventilated patients can be categorized into three main groups. First, mucoactive therapies that include expectorants and mucolytics, aimed at facilitating mucus clearance. Second, cough augmentation strategies, such as high-frequency chest wall oscillation, oscillatory positive expiratory pressure, and mechanical insufflation-exsufflation, which aid in enhancing cough mechanisms. Finally, therapies directly address inflammation and infection [2].

Conventional chest physical therapy (CCPT) is a technique used to promote airway hygiene, that involves a trained practitioner positioning the patient correctly and using a clapping technique with their hands to vibrate the thorax, aiding in the mobilization of secretions. However, CCPT has been associated with several complications, such as hypoxemia, arrhythmias, increased intracranial pressure, and carpal tunnel syndrome for the practitioners or nurses performing the therapy. Present trends indicate a rising number of patients requiring acute care hospitalization, suggesting an escalating need for supportive medical treatments, including chest physical therapy. In this context, high-frequency chest wall compressions (HFCWC) via a vibrating vest provide a mechanical alternative to CCPT. HFCWC offers potential advantages, including standardized chest physical therapy regimens and the elimination of manual administration [3]. By mimicking a 'mini-cough' through chest wall compression and relaxation, HFCWC effectively dislodges airway secretions, making it a manpower-saving substitute for CCPT [1].

High-frequency chest wall oscillation (HFCWO) is an external non-invasive respiratory modality proven effective in mobilizing airway secretions from the small peripheral airways and improving mucus rheology in patients with CF and has become an important modality in the airway clearance techniques (ACT) of this group of patients. It is a non-invasive airway clearance technique that can be used in conjunction with mechanical ventilation to improve airway clearance and reduce the risk of complications.

While chest physical therapy may offer benefits in certain clinical scenarios, such as patients with lobar atelectasis, bronchiectasis, those with impaired secretion clearance due to neuromuscular deficits, and invasively ventilated patients, recommendations for its use are limited due to the lack of well-designed, long-term trials. This chapter will discuss the use of high-frequency assisted airway clearance systems in these patients, and the concerns about their simulations use, especially the possible interaction with the ventilators settings and the safety of this strategy.

Technology of High-Frequency Assisted Airway Clearance Systems

High-Frequency Chest Wall Compression involves encasing the chest in an inflatable vest, through which a high-output compressor rapidly inflates and deflates the vest. There is a small (about 12 cm H2O) positive pressure baseline, and during inflation, this mechanism will superimpose pressure pulses on the body surface, that will range between 5–20 cm H2O during inflation, which will force the chest wall to compress and generate a short burst of expiratory flow. On deflation, the chest wall will recoil to its resting position, which will move the flow in the inspiratory direction. The Vest Airway Clearance System® operates at 2–25 Hz and generates esophageal pressure and airflow oscillations. The Vest manufacturer's states that HFCWC can generate volume changes from 17–57 mL and flows up to 1.6 L/s, that induces "mini coughs" to favor secretion mobilization. A session typically lasts 20-30 minutes and involves brief intervals at different compression frequencies, interspersed by huff coughs. HFCWC with the Vest was originally delivered with a square pressure waveform, later replaced with a sine waveform, but without any published evidence of equality of effectiveness. There are important differences between square, sine, and triangular waveforms in terms of patient volumes and flows, and that it may be best to "tune" each patient/vest combination for optimal secretion clearance. Despite HFCWC decreasing end-expiratory lung volume, its consequences debatable [4].

High-frequency Chest Wall Oscillation uses a chest cuirass, copulated to the chest wall, to generate biphasic changes in transpulmonary pressure difference. HFCWO uses a rigid chest cuirass connected to a compressor that will apply both positive and negative pressures to the body surface. This device allows the control over inspiratory and expiratory flow ratios, which theoretically may optimize mucus clearance. The Hayek oscillator, that operates at frequencies from about 1 Hz to 17 Hz, offers control of inspiratory-expiratory ratio (1:6 to 6:1) and inspiratory pressure (-70 cm H2O to 70 cm H2O). One of the preset modes is the "secretion mode," that will deliver a period of high-frequency/low-amplitude chest wall oscillation, (T1) followed by a period of high-span oscillation at low frequency (T2). T1 will last for 3 min with an inspiratory-expiratory ratio of 1:1, at 10 Hz, and with an inspiratory pressure of 12 cm H2O and an expiratory pressure of 6 cm H2O. T2 will last for 3 minutes and has an inspiratory-expiratory ratio of 5:1, a frequency of 1 Hz, an inspiratory pressure of 24 cm H2O, and an expiratory pressure of 12 cm H2O [4].

Several mechanisms have been proposed to explain the mucus transport effects of assisted airway clearance techniques. One of the most intuitive clear explanations is that mucus secretion is enhanced by air-liquid shear forces when expiratory flow surpasses the inspiratory flow, akin to a typical cough. High-frequency devices simply stack many "mini coughs" into a single spontaneous exhalation. Evidence from in vitro and in vivo experiments supports this hypothesis [4].

Understanding these mechanisms and their technology is crucial to further ensure safe and effective use of these devices, especially in ventilated patients, as this high-frequency assisted airway clearance systems may interfere with the ventilator itself.

Mechanical Ventilator - HFCWO Interactions

The advantages of HFCWC are believed to stem from its ability to enhance expiratory flows. Previous in vitro and animal research have shown that both increased expiratory flow and expiratory airflow bias are required for cephalad mucus movement [4, 5].

A key parameter for effectiveness is the ratio of peak inspiratory flow (PIF) to peak expiratory flow (PEF), with a PIF/PEF ratio of <0.9 considered to be the most effective. The optimal mucus clearance rates occur between HFCWC settings of 11–15 Hz with a peak at 13 Hz, which suggests that increased clearance of mucus is associated which reduced mucus viscosity and frequency.

The extent of HFCWC utilization among mechanically ventilated patients remains unclear, with just one report that did not distinguish the different impacts between patients who were intubated and those who were not intubated. There is a lack of comprehensive studies regarding the effects of HFCWC in patients on mechanical ventilation. High-frequency assisted airway clearance systems may be potentially unsuitable for patients on mechanical ventilation because the chest wall compression and oscillation may disrupt the flow delivery by the ventilator and triggering of additional ventilator cycles [5]. Furthermore, HFCWC may induce changes in inspiratory-expiratory flows, flow bias, and/or airway pressures (both positive and negative). These may cause a misinterpretation by the mechanical ventilator as an inspiratory trigger that leads to the delivery of additional ventilator-supported cycle and can increase the respiratory frequency and minute volume ventilation [5].

To assess the impact of HFCWC and its interaction with the ventilator, and to evaluate the effect of HFCWC on the breathing frequency, inspiratory and expiratory flow, and expiratory-inspiratory flow bias, Ntoumenopoulos et al. developed a study in an intubated and ventilated bench model and used an orally intubated mannequin that was mechanically ventilated in 5 commonly used modes of ventilation at settings that reflect current practice and HFCWC was applied via a randomized combination of oscillation frequencies and pressure settings [5].

In this study, HFCWC led to 3- to 7-fold increases in ventilator-delivered respiratory frequency during synchronized intermittent mandatory ventilation, bi-level (with pressure support), bilevel-assist, and pressure-regulated volume control modes of ventilation [4, 5]. Only in the bi-level mode without pressure support was the ventilator breathing frequency unaffected by HFCWC. During HFCWC, PIF/PEF toward an expiratory flow bias, specially at higher HFCWC pressures, only in pressure-regulated volume control and synchronized intermittent mandatory ventilation modes were PIF/PEF ratios of <0.9 generated that would facilitate secretion clearance. The bi-level mode may be the optimal mode to use with HFCWC to minimize disruption to the delivered ventilator respiratory frequency [5].

During HFCWC in synchronized intermittent mandatory ventilation - volume controlled (SIMV), bi-level with pressure support, bi-level assist, and pressure-regulated volume control (PRVC), the ventilator-delivered respiratory frequency increased significantly from baseline, supposedly due to the triggering of additional cycles from the oscillatory flow generated by HFCWC, with the ventilator set with a flow trigger of 2 L/min. The flow trigger settings commonly set for mechanical ventilation in the Intensive Care Unit (ICU) setting usually range better 1 and 4 L/min, so this 2 L/min set can be reflective of real-life conditions. In the bi-level assisted mode, no pressure support is set but additional synchronized pressure-controlled cycles were delivered due to HFCWC. HFCWC had no effect on respiratory frequency during the bi-level mode as this setting is not synchronized with any patient efforts. The additional ventilator cycles (3- to 7-fold) generated due to HFCWC seen in this study during HFCWC and SIMV, bi-level with pressure support, bi-level assist, or PRVC modes may increase minute ventilation, cause patient-ventilator asynchrony, and result in gas trapping [5].

The work by Chuang et al. reported on the impact of HFCWC in mechanically ventilated patients with pneumonia showed significant short-term increases in respiratory frequency and minute ventilation during HFCWC use (frequency set at 12 Hz). Notably, these effects were observed to return to baseline levels following the terminus of HFCWC therapy [1, 4].

In the Ntoumenopoulos et al. study, the values of PIF and PEF recorded have shown that higher HFCWC pressure settings increased the expiratory flow to a greater extent than the inspiratory flow, especially during the SIMV mode. However, prior research involving healthy subjects demonstrated that, at higher HFCWC pressure settings, there is a reduction of end-expiratory lung volume. Indeed, research has indicated that higher HFCWC pressure settings impair arterial oxygenation in acutely ill patients with pneumonia [5].

It's important to highlight that in an intubated and ventilated patient who requires frequent suctioning, HFCWC may improve ventilation, apparently due to the increased secretion clearance. A PIF/PEF of <0.9 is considered to be effective for mucus mobility in in vitro tube models. In that study, during HFCWC, effective PIF/PEF were generated by mandatory cycles only in SIMV and PRVC modes. Worth mentioning, although the PIF/PEF was still <0.9 with HFCWC during SIMV, there was a higher expiratory flow bias (at ~0.6) during baseline SIMV settings than during HFCWC. The beneficial expiratory flow bias during conventional SIMV settings probably is a result of the low lung compliance settings of the bench model as stated by other researchers, in which low lung compliance leads to an expiratory flow bias, whereas normal-to-high lung compliance leads to an inspiratory flow bias during conventional ventilation. Effective PIF/PEF < 0.9 for mucus clearance were only generated in bi-level, bilevel with pressure support, and bilevel assisted modes at higher HFCWC pressure settings. Primary constraints of this study included the use of an inert mannequin with fixed properties for airway resistance (high) and low chest wall compliance, potentially not reflecting the results seen in typical ICU patients. For this reason, these results may not be applicable to real-life ventilated patients, especially in those who are spontaneously triggering the ventilator cycles and with normal lung compliance [5].

In summary, this study concludes that ventilator mode, HFCWC oscillation frequency, and HFCWC pressure setting interfered with the ventilator respiratory frequency, inspiratory-expiratory flows, and flow bias. High ventilator respiratory frequency was recorded during HFCWC in SIMV, bi-level with pressure support, and PRVC, being HFCWC linked with triggering of additional pressure-supported cycles, whereas in bi-level assisted, additional pressure-control assisted cycles were identified. Ventilator respiratory frequency was unaltered by HFCWC in the bi-level mode, and this may be the safest mode for implementing the HFCWC in patients on mechanical ventilation, when standard chest physiotherapy is recommended but proves unsuccessful. The authors hypothesized that removing pressure support in SIMV and PRVC modes during HFCWC may allow the HFCWC to be applied without triggering additional ventilator cycles, but this demands clinical validation. The PIF/PEF was improved by HFCWC, especially at higher HFCWC pressure settings, despite an expiratory flow bias was not invariably observed in that model besides in the SIMV mode, thus, it is ambiguous when HFCWC may be indicated. In all the ventilator modes and HFCWC settings used in this ventilated model, significant changes were seen in the mechanical ventilation delivery. Potential modification of the ventilator mode or settings such as trigger setting, HFCWC oscillation, or pressure settings may be necessary to allow the safe use of HFCWC in mechanically ventilated patients [5].

Safe Use of HFCWO in Mechanically Ventilated Patients

For evaluation of the reliability of HFCWO therapy in blunt thoracic trauma patients, Anderson et al. conducted a study with 25 blunt thoracic trauma patients were HFCWO was prescribed two 15-minute sessions per day, using The Vest® Airway Clearance System that was programmed with a frequency of 10–12 Hz and a pressure of 2–3 (arbitrary unit). Physiological parameters were recorded before, during, and after each session. In this study no chest tubes, lines, drains or catheters were dislodged as a result of treatment, so it is suggested that HFCWO treatment is safe for trauma patients with lung and chest wall injuries [6].

Huang et al. conducted a study targeting to establish the effectiveness, safety, and tolerance/comfort of HFCWO after extubation in prolonged mechanical ventilation (PMV) patients [7]. This parallel-designed, randomized controlled trial enrolled 43 patients with both tracheal intubation and mechanical ventilator support continuously for at least 21 days. Upon extubation, the participants were randomly assigned to either receive HFCWO for 5 days or to standard care. The effectiveness (based on weaning success rates, daily clearance volume of sputum, serial changes in sputum coloration and chest X-ray improvement rates), safety (by physiologic parameters) and tolerance/comfort (using the Modified Borg Scale and Hamilton Anxiety Scale) of HFCWO were analyzed. There were 23 in the HFCWO group and 20 in the non-HFCWO group. The weaning success rates were 82.6% (19/23) and 85% (17/20) in the HFCWO and non-HFCWO groups, respectively ($p = 1.000$). The HFCWO group had persistently better results in daily sputum suctions and higher CXR improvement rates compared with the non-HFCWO group, and just in the HFCWO group there was a significant sputum coloration lightening. There was no significant difference neither in the tolerance/comfort nor physiologic parameters between the two groups. The authors concluded that in PMV patients, HFCWO was safe, comfortable, and effective in facilitating airway hygiene after removal of endotracheal tubes but had no positive impact on weaning success [7].

Chuang et al. conducted a study to evaluate the instantaneous changes in cardiopulmonary responses in patients on mechanical ventilation and HFCWO. This study involved 73 patients (52 men; aged 71.5 ± 13.4 years) who were intubated with mechanical ventilation for pneumonic respiratory failure, randomly assigned into 2 groups (HFCWO group, $n = 36$; and control group who received conventional chest physical therapy, $n = 37$). HFCWO was performed with a fixed protocol, while CCPT was performed using standard protocols. Both groups underwent sputum suction after each session. Changes in ventilator settings and the patients' outcomes were measured at predefined intervals and compared within groups and between groups. For detecting the immediate effects of both protocols, the measurements were carried out during a single session, usually at the initial use of HFCWO or CCPT. Changes to the initial ventilator settings during HFCWO were recorded by checking the ventilator panel before and at 5, 10, and 15 minutes during HFCWO. The assessed settings were peak airway pressure (Ppeak), positive-end expiratory pressure, respiratory rate, fraction of inspired oxygen, inspiratory time and sensitivity settings. Changes in the patients' vital signs were measured before and at 5, 10, and 15 minutes during oscillation and at 15 minutes after sputum suction. The measurement protocol for the CCPT group was the same as for the HFCWO group, except that no measurements were taken at 5 or 10 minutes during percussion, as its logistics was not possible for a single nurse. The primary outcome was differences in the Ppeak between baseline and 15 minutes after suction. The secondary outcome was differences in the other cardiopulmonary variables between baseline and 15 minutes after suction. The results of this study have shown that oscillation did not affect the ventilator settings (all $p > 0.05$). The mean airway pressure, respiratory frequency, and rapid shallow breathing index increased, and the tidal volume and SpO2 decreased (all $p < 0.05$). After sputum suction, the Ppeak and minute ventilation decreased (all $p < 0.05$). The HFCWO group had a lower tidal volume and SpO2 at the end of oscillation, and lower Ppeak and tidal volume after sputum suction than the CCPT group. The authors conclude that HFCWO affects breathing pattern and SpO2 but not ventilator settings, whereas CCPT maintains a steadier condition. After sputum suction, HFCWO slightly improved Ppeak compared to CCPT, suggesting that the study extends the indications of HFCWO for these patients in intensive care unit [1].

Conclusion

As detailed in this chapter, there is some diverging evidence on the impact of high-frequency assisted airway clearance systems on the mechanical ventilator settings, which highlights the importance of evaluating these interactions, to ensure safe and effective use of these devices in mechanically ventilated patients. Nevertheless, despite its interaction with the ventilator, these devices seem to be safe and do improve airway hygiene in ventilated patients.

More clinical trials and real-life studies will further help the clinicians to feel comfortable to use these interventions, and more experience will come with more practice in this area.

Key Messages

1. Critically ill patients often experience impaired cough reflex and ineffective mucociliary clearance due to sedation, inadequate humidification, and other key factors related to mechanical ventilation. Implementing airway clearance strategies, such as manual hyperinflation and appropriate suctioning techniques, is essential to mitigate these issues.
2. HFCWC offers potential advantages over conventional chest physical therapy, providing standardized regimens and eliminating the need for manual administration. It effectively dislodges airway secretions, making it a manpower-saving substitute for chest physiotherapy.
3. The effectiveness of HFCWC depends on various factors such as oscillation frequency and pressure settings. While it can improve mucus clearance, it may interfere with ventilator settings and trigger additional cycles, potentially causing patient-ventilator asynchrony and gas trapping.
4. Studies suggest that HFCWO is safe and effective in facilitating airway hygiene in mechanically ventilated patients, leading to improvements in sputum clearance and chest X-ray findings. However, it may affect breathing patterns and oxygen saturation, necessitating careful monitoring during use.

References

[1] Chuang ML, Chou YL, Lee CY, Huang SF. Instantaneous responses to high-frequency chest wall oscillation in patients with acute pneumonic respiratory failure receiving mechanical ventilation: A randomized controlled study. *Medicine (Baltimore)* 2017 Mar;96(9):e5912.
[2] Goetz RL, Vijaykumar K, Solomon GM. Mucus Clearance Strategies in Mechanically Ventilated Patients. *Frontiers in Physiology* 2022 Mar;13:834716.
[3] Lin YP, Tung HH, Wang TJ. Comparative Study of High-frequency Chest Wall Oscillation and Traditional Chest Physical Therapy in Intensive Care Unit Patients. *Journal of Comprehensive Nursing Research and Care* 2017 Nov;2:115.

[4] Chatburn RL. High-frequency assisted airway clearance. *Respiratory Care* 2007 Sep;52(9):1224-35; discussion 1235-7.
[5] Ntoumenopoulos G, Jones A, Koutoumanou E, Shannon H. The Impact of High-Frequency Chest-Wall Compression on Mechanical Ventilation Delivery and Flow Bias. *Respiratory Care* 2023 Aug;69(1):respcare.10932.
[6] Anderson CA, Palmer CA, Ney AL, Becker B, Schaffel SD, Quickel RR. Evaluation of the safety of high-frequency chest wall oscillation (HFCWO) therapy in blunt thoracic trauma patients. *Journal of Trauma Management & Outcomes* 2008 Oct;6;2(1):8.
[7] Huang WC, Wu PC, Chen CJ, Cheng YH, Shih SJ, Chen HC, Wu CL. High-frequency chest wall oscillation in prolonged mechanical ventilation patients: a randomized controlled trial. *The Clinical Respiratory Journal* 2016 May;10(3):272-81.

Chapter 8

High-Frequency Chest Wall Oscillation Therapy in the Critically Ill: Summary and Key Practical Approaches

Ahmad Mohammad Alessa[1],*
and Antonio M. Esquinas[2], MD

[1]King Abdullah Medical City, Makkah, Saudi Arabia
[2]Intensive Care Unit, Hospital Morales Meseguer, Murcia, Spain

Abstract

This chapter primarily summarizes the concepts discussed in the other chapters, focusing on high-frequency chest wall oscillation (HFCWO). HFCWO is defined as a chest physical therapy that involves using an inflatable vest to loosen and thin mucus so that it can be easily coughed up or eliminated from the airway. The machine has two pieces: an air-pulse generator and an inflatable vest, with the former being used for pumping air into the latter. HFCWO mobilizes pulmonary secretions through the air-liquid interaction. Timely diagnosis and use of HFCWO to clear the airways can significantly reduce mortality and morbidity.

Keywords: high-frequency chest wall oscillation, critically ill, mechanical ventilation

---

* Corresponding Author's Email: alessa.a@kamc.med.sa.

In: High-frequency Chest Wall Oscillation Therapy in Critical Ill Patients
Editor: Antonio M. Esquinas
ISBN: 979-8-89530-264-4
© 2025 Nova Science Publishers, Inc.

Introduction

HFCWO pressure and frequency vary, and patients can adjust the settings to their preferences; even though the standard prescription of high-frequency HFCWO has been 30 minutes twice daily and has been used for more than two decades, it is suggested that patients have varying needs and tolerance levels [1]. Thus, clinical guidance should be invited to ensure the most appropriate settings are used. The settings should be reevaluated frequently to ensure recovery is considered in determining the most suitable setting for a patient [1].

Because of the nature of HFCWO therapy, it has been observed to be effective in handling multiple respiratory health conditions. All the health conditions for adults and children that can be managed or prevented using HFCWO benefit from the extent to which the therapy enhances healthy air circulation and limits the likeliness of infection by accumulating mucus on the airway walls. HFCWO can effectively manage some conditions so they do not escalate to more significant concerns such as pneumonia. It is also used to transition from long-term dependence on physical ventilation after prolonged illness.

Rationale

High-frequency chest wall oscillation (HFCWO) is a type of chest physical therapy involving an inflatable vest attached to a high-frequency vibration machine. As the chest vibrates, the chest loosens and thins mucus. The process was first described by Khoo et al. [1]. HFCWO has, over the years, been used to manage various chest-related health conditions, including asthma. However, the discovery of HFCWO's effectiveness in managing multiple conditions did not happen instantaneously.

HFCWO oscillates at the speed of 180 to 600 cycles per minute. The machine has two parts: an air-pulse generator and an inflatable vest. The vest applies small-volume expiratory pulses on the external chest wall, leading to high-velocity expiratory airflow that drives secretion because of the force created by Leemans et al. [2]. The latter is connected to a generator by horses. Air from the generator is sent through the horse, causing rapid inflation and deflation in the vest at a rate that might get as high as 20 times each second. Inflation and deflation create a type of pressure that is similar to what happens when someone claps. The resultant vibration separates mucus from the airway and helps move it into the large airways. This is why using the vest takes someone five minutes before they begin to cough or huff cough because of the urge to clear the throat. The session is supposed to take between 20 and 30 minutes. It can be self-administered because of the ease of the physics underlying the functioning of HFCWO.

HFCWO mobilizes pulmonary secretions primarily by air-liquid interaction. When HFCWO is at work, chest compression is inducted, leading to rapid air movement into and out of the lung. The vibration on the chest wall leads to a transient increase in airflow into the lungs, which increases mucus mobility and gas-liquid interactions. The flow bias characterized by whether inspiration or expiration dominates the airways determines whether the mucus moves upwards or downwards. Empirical evidence confirms that oscillation frequency and the synchronized effects of flow bias are directly proportional to mucus clearance. The effects are evident in the central and peripheral lung regions. The primary benefit of HFCWO is the clearance of the airways. Thus, it is appropriate for various complications related to the accumulation of mucus in the respiratory system without exclusively focusing on the airways. The device is practical regarding the accumulation of mucus in the airways as it breaks up the mucus and brings it to the upper airways, where it can either be coughed out or removed. When successfully used, HFCWO can improve lung functioning with time, reducing chest infections. Also, HFCWO can lessen the need for antibiotics and hospital admissions and readmissions.

Timely diagnosis and use of airway clearance can reduce mortality and morbidity. The intention of implementing airway clearance is to minimize the damage to the airway by stopping a vicious cycle of bacterial infection and inflammation. It is also a way of reducing pulmonary exacerbations and hospitalizations. As a result, the treatment recipients see their quality of life improve. It is also considered a cornerstone in mitigating airway infection, obstruction, and inflammation associated with some ailments, such as bronchiectasis [3]. However, the benefits should not be assumed to be limited to such conditions.

Methodology

To understand how HFCWO works, there is often the need to know the equipment involved. HFCWO is a device that uses an air compressor and a vest with inflatable bladders linked to the compressor by a large but flexible tube [4]. The compressor pumps air into the vest at a frequency that varies depending on the settings. Thus, the pressure that is exerted on the vest also varies. The simplicity of the equipment used in this therapy makes it possible for the treatment to be self-administered at the patient's convenience. With few components, the equipment also has high mobility and can be used in different settings and by patients with varying lifestyles.

The variance in HFCWO pressure and frequency indicates that users can always set these parameters based on their needs. However, this is only possible after practical guidance. The frequency of use of the device ranges from two to 25 [5]. Lower-pressure/mid-frequency settings are the most commonly used option in implementing HFCWO to clear the airway [6]. However, a frequency adjustment, which also impacts the amount of pressure exerted, is possible when the typical setting does not meet a patient's needs for more than 20 years; the standard prescription of high-frequency HFCWO has been 30 minutes twice daily [7]. This usage history is primarily based on the similarity of the manuals users get that guide them on how to use the device. However, such guidance might not always be relevant to what patients need. However, the long-term effectiveness of the therapy highly depends on how the users learn to balance the duration of exposure and the intensity so that they get a combination that matches their needs [7]. The variances might depend on differences in attributes such as personal tolerance and lifestyle. Even though no patient can experience the benefits of HFCWO, consistency needs to be practiced. However, not all patients have been observed to need the 30-minute therapy rule. Thus, a patient-centered approach can only be achieved if flexibility is introduced in the prescription of HFCWO therapy.

Even though self-administration of HFCWO is possible, clinical monitoring is encouraged. Having observed that there is no one-fit-all prescription for HFCWO therapy, clinicians should be involved in introducing flexible prescriptions depending on the needs of individual patients [7]. Patients should not assume that they will get what they need from the high-frequency HFCWO, which has been 30 30-minute, twice-each-day prescription that has been considered standard for more than 20 years. The manufacturers of the devices often use the frequency for all patients without considering variances in aspects such as tolerance and need. Thus, patients should involve clinicians in monitoring their response to HFCWO therapy so that they find the appropriate combination of frequency and pressure. Patient-centered treatment can be achieved by actively monitoring HFCWO therapy.

Clinical Applications

HFCWO Adult Critical Care Applications

The difference between noninvasive and invasive ventilation can highlight how HFCWO therapy enhances health outcomes in clinical settings. The interface distinguishes the two forms of ventilation between the patient and the ventilator. Noninvasive ventilation (NIV) is an intervention that does not involve using an artificial airway [8]. HFCWO therapy falls under this category because of the lack of intrusion; HFCWO therapy is considered safe. Because of this nature, self-administration is allowed when used in most contexts. However, the need for clinical monitoring and guidance should not be overlooked for the effectiveness and optimization of patient experiences. Invasive mechanical ventilation provides a unique experience for the patient and is used in settings different from those in which HFCWO therapy is considered necessary. Invasive mechanical ventilation entails delivering positive pressure to the lungs through a tracheostomy or endotracheal tube. When a patient undergoes invasive mechanical ventilation, a predetermined mixture of oxygen and other gases is used to force into the patient's central airway, from where it flows into the alveoli [9]. During the lung inflation, there is a simultaneous increase in the intra-alveolar pressure. The ventilator stops forcing air into the central airways when it gets a termination signal from attaining the desired pressure or flow.

The clinical application of HFCWO is best understood in the context of nasal high-flow oxygen. According to empirical evidence, nasal high-flow oxygen reduces the amount of nasopharyngeal airway resistance. By doing so, the rate of oxygenation and ventilation are improved [10]. HFCWO is related to the flow of oxygen because of the extent to which it frees the airway of mucus, making it possible for a sufficient flow of oxygen to the lungs.

Some patients might need long-term ventilation due to their respiratory constraints and health conditions. However, there comes a time when they are weaning from physical ventilation, which is necessary. Ventilator weaning should be strategic and progressive [11]. The process should also be tailored to the individual needs of each patient. For example, in HFCWO, there is no one-fit-all approach to achieving the goals of ventilation weaning [12]. Noninvasive ventilation is among the measures taken to facilitate weaning from prolonged mechanical ventilation.

HFCWO can be used to prevent and treat extubation respiratory failure. Even though coughing might be sufficient for expectoration for patients suffering from pneumonia, it is impractical for acute pneumonic patients with respiratory failure to receive mechanical ventilation, endotracheal intubation, and sedation [13]. HFCWO can be used in managing and preventing respiratory failure because of the self-propagating mucus production cycle, and the airway damages that might lead to chronic infections and inflammations have the same implications as those associated with respiratory failure patients, especially those that need mechanical ventilation [14]. It should not be forgotten that excessive trachea-bronchial secretions can lead to extubation failure, another situation in which HFCWO can be used for intervention. HFCWO has also been effective, safe, and comfortable for prolonged mechanical ventilation (PMV) patients, especially considering the need to maintain high hygiene levels after the endotracheal tubes are removed. A recent study observed that although HFCWO was associated with high costs, its inclusion increased the effectiveness in preventing lung atelectasis or hospital-acquired pneumonia in a way that routine pulmonary rehabilitation does not [15]. Thus, HFCWO not only facilitates the management of respiratory failure but also contributes to its prevention.

HFCWO therapy is among the recommendations for treating chronic obstructive pulmonary disorders (COPD) and other conditions such as cystic fibrosis, bronchiectasis, and other impaired breathing issues. HFCWO provides patients with the possibility of managing their conditions. HFCWO has also been observed to be well-tailored to the care needs of adults hospitalized for COPD and acute asthma, especially considering its effectiveness in reducing dyspnea [16]. The instrument is scalable enough to address the varying experiences and needs of patients suffering from these conditions. With the proper clinical guidance, patients can always understand the settings that optimize their experiences.

HFCWO therapy is also effective for individuals with neuromuscular pulmonary disorders. People with this condition have difficulty in clearing pulmonary secretions, a factor that puts them at risk of respiratory failure and pneumonia [17]. HFCWO therapy can help such individuals clear their secretions. This intervention has been proven adequate as a secretion mobilization technique that mobilizes the mucus in the peripheral airways to ease removal. HFCWO helps loosen and thin the mucus so it is easily separated from the airway walls. However, the frequency and intensity of the clearance of the airways should be customized for patients with such a condition. Also, regular reevaluation is proposed during the treatment. This is because there might be a need to reduce the intensity and frequency as a patient gets better.

HFCWO is one of the techniques that can be used to prevent ventilator-associated pneumonia (VAP). Preventing VAP should be done by understanding the risk factors. HFCWO serves this purpose by doing what it does best: clearing the airways. The therapeutic benefits of this therapy are based on the understanding that it presents the accumulation of mucus on the airway walls. When such an action is undertaken consistently, there is a resultant improvement in respiratory health and a decline in the likeliness of having VAP. Noninvasive ventilation approaches have also been highlighted as prevention strategies for reducing the likelihood of ventilator exposure, a factor that is considered a risk factor for VAP. Thus, one would instead use HFCWO than wait for ventilator exposure.

Pediatric Mechanically Ill Patients

HFCWO applies in cystic fibrosis exacerbations. Cystic fibrosis exacerbations are characterized by chronic respiratory infections, leading to an increased risk of lung function loss. To understand the severity of being in such a situation, the focus should be on the role lungs play in the human body. According to a recent study, HFCWO can be used in managing the symptoms of cystic fibrosis exacerbations, as there is an almost immediate improvement in lung function after an instance of HFCWO administration [18]. Such an outcome proves a correlation between lung health and clarity of the airways. One of the possible explanations is that the latter impacts the effective movement of oxygen and carbon dioxide into and out of the lungs.

HFCWO can be manageable in the management of non-cystic fibrosis. Non-cystic fibrosis is a condition that is characterized by inflammation of the lung, often as a result of respiratory infections and persistent coughing. HFCWO is a commonly accepted treatment for non-cystic fibrosis because of its superiority in effectiveness compared to the available alternatives [18]. Such an observation is based on the responses from patients who have used HFCWO. It helps manage non-cystic fibrosis by eliminating excessive mucus on the airway mall, thus reducing the likeliness of any infections and eventually protecting the lungs from inflammation that might result from such a situation.

Due to the nature of HFCWO, HFO, and HCW, there are numerous possibilities for using them in a clinical context. This therapy approach focuses on the constant mucus coating on the airway walls, which should be cleared to allow for proper intake and expulsion of air in and out of the body. An otherwise environment lays an individual open to a set of multiple conditions. As such, HFCWO appropriately addresses the number of diseases described above and can also be used to prevent them. However, HFCWO is safe and can be easily used, as evidenced by the provision for inclusive and noninvasive self-administration. However, patients should always engage clinical professionals in getting the context that adequately suits their needs. As stated above, there is no specific working environment where this method can be applied to different conductions.

Conclusion

In conclusion, high-frequency chest wall oscillation treatment is a feasible and accessible model for addressing many respiratory conditions in patients in critical condition. Thus, by facilitating airway clearance, HFCWO attenuates the possibilities of pneumonia and ventilator-associated pneumonia, positively impacting lung performance. Due to its noninvasive characteristics and the fact that it can fine tune chosen patient parameters to be matched, it is a valuable aid in patient therapy and enhancing respiratory health. However, clinical direction and supervision establish the ideal practical range of HFCWO treatment and patients' potential outcomes in the critical care environment. Moreover, by showing marked improvement in the patient's quality of life, the outcomes prove that a patient-centered approach to HFCWO treatment is practical. Ad hoc therapy may be necessary since patient tolerance, need for treatment, and response varies. Clinical knowledge, therefore, results in a positive and active approach to respiratory care by altering the treatment variables to enhance both effectiveness and patient comfort. Besides, the role of HFCWO is not limited to providing comfort for further primary symptoms; it is the key to reducing exacerbations, facilitating the weaning process in patients who need ventilatory support, and increasing their overall outcomes. This makes it financially impactful by having the capacity to lower hospitalization and readmission apart from curtailing healthcare utilization. Employing such ideas as the HFCWO therapy during the critical care processes as healthcare technologies would assist in enhancing the sufferance of patients through increased competencies and optimality. Therefore, more studies are needed concerning its impacts in the long run, proper usage patterns, and application within different routes of

High-Frequency Chest Wall Oscillation Therapy in the Critically Ill

multidisciplinary therapeutic. Thus, HFCWO treatment remains the primary treatment for total respiratory disease in critically ill patients. Hence, it is clear that HFCWO can enhance lung function, facilitate airway clearance, and lower issues, proving the potential of technology in delivering critical care treatment. Recognizing its potential and furthering its application would undoubtedly help offer patients better outcomes and a brighter future for individuals needing necessary treatment interventions.

Key Messages

1. High-frequency chest wall oscillation (HFCWO) therapy is an effective airway clearance technique for critically ill patients, facilitating the removal of mucus and improving lung function.
2. HFCWO therapy varies in pressure and frequency, and patients should adjust settings based on individual needs, with clinical guidance recommended for optimal results.
3. HFCWO therapy is beneficial for managing various respiratory conditions, including COPD, cystic fibrosis exacerbations, and neuromuscular pulmonary disorders.
4. Timely diagnosis and use of HFCWO can reduce mortality and morbidity by preventing complications such as pneumonia and ventilator-associated pneumonia.
5. HFCWO therapy complements ventilator weaning strategies and can prevent extubation respiratory failure by facilitating secretion mobilization.
6. Noninvasive nature of HFCWO therapy makes it safe for self-administration, but clinical monitoring is essential for effectiveness and patient optimization.
7. In pediatric mechanically ill patients, HFCWO effectively manages cystic fibrosis exacerbations and non-cystic fibrosis conditions by improving lung function and reducing infection risk.
8. HFCWO therapy is scalable and adaptable to individual patient needs, contributing to enhanced respiratory health outcomes and improved quality of life.
9. The prevention of ventilator-associated pneumonia can be achieved through consistent use of HFCWO, reducing the accumulation of mucus on airway walls.

10. The versatility and ease of use of HFCWO therapy make it a valuable tool in critical care settings for adult and pediatric patients.

References

[1] Khoo, M. C., Ye, T. H., & Tran, N. H. Lung pressures and gas transport during high-frequency airway and chest wall oscillation Journal *of Applied Physiology* 1989. *67*(3), 985-992.

[2] Leemans, G., Belmans, D., Van Holsbeke, C., Becker, B., Vissers, D., Ides, K., & Van Hoorenbeeck, K. The effectiveness of a mobile high-frequency chest wall oscillation (HFCWO) device for airway clearance. *Pediatric Pulmonology* 2020. 55(8), 1984-1992.

[3] Daynes, E. Symptom Management of Chronic Obstructive Pulmonary Disease Using High-Frequency Airway Oscillations (Doctoral dissertation, University of Leicester) 2020.

[4] Leelarungrayub, J., Pinkaew, D., Wonglangka, K., Eungpinichpong, W., & Klaphajone, J. Short-term pulmonary rehabilitation for a female patient with chronic scleroderma under single-case research design Clinical Medicine Insights: Circulatory, Respiratory and Pulmonary Medicine 2016. 10, CCRPM-S40050.

[5] Chatburn, R. L. High-frequency assisted airway clearance: high-frequency chest-wall oscillation and compression are two methods used for airway clearance, but there may be no benefit except for patience preference RT for Decision Makers in Respiratory Care 2008. 21(8), 30-34.

[6] Kempainen, R. R., Milla, C., Dunitz, J., Savik, K., Hazelwood, A., Williams, C. Comparison of settings used for high-frequency chest-wall compression in cystic fibrosis Respiratory *care* 2010, 55(6), 695-701.

[7] Pandya, P. K., Hansen, G., Daignault, S., Kasper, B., & Parada, N. A. Adaptive High-Frequency Chest Wall Oscillation (HFCWO) Therapy for Maximum Patient Adherence: A Patient-Centered Approach. *Respiratory Therapy*, 2019. 14(4), 68-70.

[8] Popowicz, P., & Leonard, K. Noninvasive ventilation and oxygenation strategies. *Surgical Clinics* 2022. 102(1), 149-157.

[9] Hyzy, R. C., & McSparron, J. I. Overview of initiating invasive mechanical ventilation in adults in the intensive care unit UpToDate *2021*.

[10] Lewins, K., Morrissey, A. M., Remorini, C., Castro, M. D. P., Noonan, M., Teves, L., & Niranjan, V. The "knock-on" effects of COVID-19 on healthcare services In Caring on the Frontline during COVID-19: Contributions from Rapid Qualitative Research (pp. 253-291) Singapore: Springer Singapore. 2022.

[11] Ambrosino, N., & Vitacca, M. The patient needing prolonged mechanical ventilation: a narrative review Multidisciplinary *respiratory medicine* 2018. *13*(1), 1-10.

[12] Ceriana, P., Nava, S., Vitacca, M., Carlucci, A., Paneroni, M., Schreiber, A., Ambrosino, N. Noninvasive ventilation during weaning from prolonged mechanical ventilation. *Pulmonology* 2019. *25*(6), 328-333.

[13] Chuang, M. L., Chou, Y. L., Lee, C. Y. Huang, S. F. Instantaneous responses to high-frequency chest wall oscillation in patients with acute pneumonic respiratory failure receiving mechanical ventilation: A randomized controlled study. *Medicine* 2017. *96*(9).

[14] Goetz, R. L., Vijaykumar, K., & Solomon, G. M. Mucus clearance strategies in mechanically ventilated patients. *Frontiers in Physiology* 2022. *13*, 834716.

[15] Kuyrukluyildiz, U., Binici, O., Kupeli, İ., Erturk, N., Gulhan, B., Akyol, F., & Karabakan, G. What is the best pulmonary physiotherapy method in ICU?. *Canadian Respiratory Journal 2016.* 2016:2016:4752467.

[16] Mahajan, A. K., Diette, G. B., Hatipoğlu, U., Bilderback, A., Ridge, A., Harris, V. W. High-frequency chest wall oscillation for asthma and chronic obstructive pulmonary disease exacerbations: a randomized sham-controlled clinical trial. *Respiratory research.* 2011 Sep 10;12(1):120.

[17] Lechtzin, N., Wolfe, L. F., & Frick, K. D. The impact of high-frequency chest wall oscillation on healthcare use in patients with neuromuscular diseases. *Annals of the American Thoracic Society* 2016. *13*(6), 904-909.

[18] Barto, T. L., Maselli, D. J., Daignault, S., Stiglich, J., Porter, J., Kraemer, C. Real-life experience with high-frequency chest wall oscillation vest therapy in adults with non-cystic fibrosis bronchiectasis Therapeutic advances in respiratory disease. 2020 14, 1753466620932508.

Chapter 9

High-Frequency Chest Wall Oscillation and Nasal High Flow Oxygen

Francisco Neri[*], MD
Pulmonology Department, Hospital Beatriz Ângelo, Loures, Portugal

Abstract

High-flow nasal cannula therapy (HFNC), delivering heated and humidified oxygen offers reliable FiO2 control, reducing dead space and leaks. Beneficial in various clinical scenarios, HFNC improves patient comfort, oxygenation, and reduces respiratory complications. In acute hypoxemic respiratory failure, it outperforms conventional oxygen therapy, potentially preventing intubation. HFNC's advantages extends to obstructive airway diseases, optimizing mucociliary clearance. Defective mucociliary clearance elevates respiratory risks, emphasizing the importance of HFNC. Intensive care unit patients face increased respiratory infection risks due to impaired secretion clearance. Kinesiotherapy, including incorporation of high-frequency chest wall oscillation (HFCWO), aids mucociliary clearance by inducing mucolytic and accelerating clearance, demonstrating safety and effectiveness. Theoretical benefits emerge when combining HFNC with HFCWO, promoting optimal mucociliary clearance. An integrated strategy, blending ventilation modalities like HFNC and HFCWO with secretion drainage, emerges. This approach, unexplored in adults, may mitigate non-invasive ventilation failure, reducing intubation risks. HFNC and HFCWO offer substantial respiratory benefits individually. The theoretical synergy between these modalities presents an intriguing avenue for optimizing mucociliary clearance. An integrated strategy,

---

[*] Corresponding Author's Email: f.neri.93@gmail.com.

In: High-frequency Chest Wall Oscillation Therapy in Critical Ill Patients
Editor: Antonio M. Esquinas
ISBN: 979-8-89530-264-4
© 2025 Nova Science Publishers, Inc.

combining ventilation and clearance techniques, holds promise in reducing the risk of non-invasive ventilation failure in adult patients, emphasizing the need for further research.

Keywords: high flow nasal cannula therapy, airway secretions, critical care, mechanical ventilation, high-frequency chest wall oscillation

Introduction

High flow nasal cannula (HFNC) therapy is an oxygen supply system that's capable of delivering heated and 100% humidified oxygen at a flow rate of up to 60 liters per minute [1]. In contrast to low flow nasal cannula, where an open system of supplementation is observed and therefore contributes to high levels of leaking air around the oxygen source, only delivering 4 to 6 liters per minute of oxygen (if a traditional nasal cannula is used) that corresponds to a FiO2 of approximately 0.37 to 0.45, HFNC therapy allows for more reliable control of the delivered FiO2 to the patient and reduces dead space and existing leaks [1, 2].

Its benefits are well-established, ranging from clinical advantages such as patient comfort and ease of use to physiological benefits like increased oxygenation, alveolar recruitment, heating, and humidification of the delivered air, reduced dead space, and ease in secretion clearance. Recent studies also indicate its potential to prevent decline in lung function and decrease the rate of endotracheal intubations [1, 2].

In terms of adult intensive care, the application of HFNC has been suggested for various clinical situations, with particular utility in acute hypoxemic respiratory failure. Studies show that, when compared to conventional oxygen therapy, HFNC therapy has demonstrated superiority by matching the inspiratory demand of hypoxemic patients, allowing for a reliable delivery of FiO2 up to 100%. Simultaneously, it provides a low level of positive end-expiratory pressure (PEEP) in the upper airways, facilitating alveolar recruitment. Although its impact on mortality is low, this type of therapy is considered beneficial for high-risk patients for intubation, and in some cases, it may obviate the need for intubation. In patients with progressive or moderate to severe acute respiratory failure (PaO2/FiO2 ratio <= 200 mmHg), non-invasive ventilation (NIV) has a higher failure rate, and some authors recommend a trial of HFNC in these patients. Furthermore, the superiority of HFNC over conventional oxygen therapy has been demonstrated in patients requiring NIV pauses, for example those in need of feeding. Both HFNC and NIV have shown efficacy in high-risk patients for respiratory complications in postoperative extubation [1].

Regarding acute hypercapnic respiratory failure, the latest guidelines recommend the initial use of NIV over HFNC. However, some other studies indicate that both modalities can be beneficial in this type of respiratory failure [1].

The fact that this type of therapy allows for the delivery of humidified and heated oxygen to the patient has advantages in eliminating secretions from the respiratory tract. The mucociliary transport system, extending from bronchioles to the nasopharynx, acts as a defense mechanism in which contaminants trapped in the airway are transported out. This physiological system is most effective at a normal body temperature and with 100% relative humidity, being highly sensitive to changes in these conditions [2]. In situations of low humidity and decreased airway temperature below normal, there is a change in the viscosity of respiratory secretions, bronchoconstriction can occur and both ciliary beat frequency and mucociliary clearance speed are reduced. In conventional low-flow nasal cannula oxygen therapy systems, oxygen is supplied at low temperatures and with low relative humidity, altering the properties of respiratory mucus and causing bronchoconstriction. This effect becomes more pronounced in patients with heightened sensitivity, such as those with asthma or COPD [2]. Defective mucociliary clearance reduces pulmonary compliance, increases airway resistance, raises the workload on respiratory muscles, and is associated with the risk of mucus plug formation, alveolar de-recruitment, and airway infection. In patients with COPD or bronchiectasis, where chronic mucus hyper-secretion occurs, predisposing them to chronic bacterial colonization, respiratory infections, decline in lung function, and an increased risk of hospitalization, these deleterious effects of conventional oxygen therapy can be more pronounced. Studies demonstrate that the inhalation of hyper-humidified air at temperatures around 37°C in patients with obstructive airway diseases has beneficial effects for the reasons already mentioned [2].

Patients admitted to intensive care units have a higher rate of post-extubation respiratory infections due to the inability to clear secretions. Whether due to inhibited reflexes or intubation-related myopathy, patients require kinesiotherapy techniques to strengthen weakened muscles and aid in the elimination of accumulated secretions, allowing for complete mucociliary clearance. These techniques may involve respiratory kinesiotherapy exercises, cough-assist devices, or other devices designed to facilitate the elimination of secretions.

High-frequency chest wall oscillation (HFCWO) therapy has shown benefits in patients admitted to intensive care units. By applying vibrations using a chest vest, it allows for rapid air movement, inducing mucolytic and increasing mucociliary clearance [2]. It has been suggested that this type of therapy be incorporated into kinesiotherapy techniques, administered routinely to hospitalized patients to reduce discomfort. Some studies demonstrate that its use is safe, comfortable, and effective in eliminating bronchial secretions [3]. When used twice daily, it improves oxygenation and static lung compliance, allowing for better secretion clearance compared to its once-daily use [4].

In theoretical terms, the combination of HFNC with HFCWO has its advantages. By allowing humidification and the heating of oxygen supplied to the patient, there is greater ease in eliminating secretions from the respiratory tract. Combining secretion clearance techniques, such as the application of HFCWO to the patient, will allow for synergy between the two methods, optimizing mucociliary clearance in the patient admitted to the intensive care unit.

There are no available studies regarding the simultaneous use of the two procedures described above. Some reports demonstrate their utility in premature newborn models where, in vitro, the combination of improved CO_2 clearance and reduced pressure delivery proved to be a useful improvement in the respiratory care of infants in respiratory distress [5]. No studies have been conducted in adults comparing the use of HFCWO in patients with and without HFNC. However, an integrated strategy combining various ventilation modalities with secretion drainage techniques, including HFCWO, appears to be the most promising approach to reduce the risk of non-invasive ventilation failure and the subsequent need for intubation [6].

In summary, HFCWO therapy, administered through a chest vest, has demonstrated benefits in intensive care unit patients by inducing mucolytic and enhancing mucociliary clearance. Its incorporation into kinesiotherapy techniques is suggested for routine administration in hospitalized patients to alleviate discomfort. The theoretical combination of HFCWO with HFNC presents advantages, facilitating secretion elimination through oxygen humidification and heating. Although no studies have investigated the simultaneous use of these procedures in adults, reports highlight their utility in premature newborn models.

Conclusion

Overall, an integrated strategy combining various ventilation modalities, including HFNC, with secretion drainage techniques such as HFCWO emerges as a promising approach to reduce the risk of non-invasive ventilation failure and the subsequent need for intubation in adults.

Key Messages

1. HFNC Advantages: HFNC therapy provides reliable control of inspired oxygen levels, reducing dead space and leakage, offering benefits in patient comfort and physiological outcomes.
2. Clinical Utility: HFNC demonstrates superiority in acute hypoxemic respiratory failure, surpassing conventional oxygen therapy, potentially preventing the need for endotracheal intubation in high-risk patients.
3. Mucociliary Clearance: HFNC, combined with techniques like HFCWO, proves effective in enhancing mucociliary clearance, vital for patients facing respiratory challenges, such as those in intensive care units.
4. Integrated Strategy: The theoretical combination of HFNC with HFCWO suggests synergistic advantages in optimizing mucociliary clearance. While studies on simultaneous use in adults are lacking, an integrated approach incorporating various ventilation modalities shows promise in reducing non-invasive ventilation failure risks.
5. Research Gaps: Despite the theoretical benefits, there is a notable lack of studies on the simultaneous use of HFNC and HFCWO in adults. The potential benefits of an integrated strategy combining these modalities require further exploration through dedicated research in adult populations.

References

[1] Oczkowski S., Ergan B., Bos L., Chatwin M., Ferrer M., Gregoretti C., Heunks L., Frat J., Longhini F., Nava S., Navalesi P., Uğurlu A., Pisani L., Renda T., Thille A., Winck J., Windisch W., Tonia T., Boyd J., Sotgiu G., Scala R. 2022. ERS clinical

practice guidelines: high-flow nasal cannula in acute respiratory failure. *European Respiratory Journal* 2022, 59 (4) 2101574.

[2] D'Cruz, R. F., Hart, N., Kaltsakas, G. High-flow therapy: physiological effects and clinical applications. *Breathe* 2020. 16(4), 200224.

[3] Huang, W. C., Wu, P. C., Chen, C. J., Cheng, Y. H., Shih, S. J., Chen, H. C., Wu, C. L. High-frequency chest wall oscillation in prolonged mechanical ventilation patients: a randomized controlled trial. *The clinical respiratory journal* 2016. 10(3), 272–281.

[4] Ge, J., Ye, Y., Tan, Y., Liu, F., Jiang, Y., Lu, J. High-frequency chest wall oscillation multiple times daily can better reduce the loss of pulmonary surfactant and improve lung compliance in mechanically ventilated patients. *Heart & lung : the journal of critical care* 2023. 61, 114–119.

[5] Rub, D. M., Sivieri, E. M., Abbasi, S., Eichenwald, E. Effect of high-frequency oscillation on pressure delivered by high flow nasal cannula in a premature infant lung model. *Pediatric pulmonology* 2019; 54(11), 1860–1865.

[6] Scala, R., Pisani, L. Noninvasive ventilation in acute respiratory failure: which recipe for success? *European respiratory review* : an official journal of the European Respiratory Society 2018. 27(149), 180029.

Chapter 10

Weaning from Mechanical Ventilation and Pulmonary Rehabilitation

Berkan Basançelebi[*]
Department of Electroneurophysiology, Vocational School, Istanbul Medipol University, Istanbul, Turkey

Abstract

Technological advancements in healthcare introduce new methods and strategies. High-frequency devices represent innovative approaches in pulmonary rehabilitation and critical care. While high-frequency chest wall oscillation (HFCWO) is primarily used in patients with cystic fibrosis, it also has various other applications. It contributes airway clearance on the chest wall, affecting inspiratory and expiratory flow dynamics.

Mechanical ventilation dependence is an undesirable outcome in clinical management as it increases healthcare workload and costs. Numerous studies are focused on reducing this dependence. HFCWO can be effectively utilized in weaning, liberation from mechanical ventilation, and pulmonary rehabilitation to maintain airway clearance, beyond its primary use in cystic fibrosis.

This chapter aims to present the role of the high-frequency chest wall oscillation in mechanical ventilator dependence and weaning, and its potential benefits in pulmonary rehabilitation from a different perspective.

Keywords: high-frequency chest wall oscillation, high-frequency chest wall compression, mechanical ventilation, weaning, pulmonary rehabilitation

---

[*] Corresponding Author's Email: berkanbasancelebi@gmail.com.

In: High-frequency Chest Wall Oscillation Therapy in Critical Ill Patients
Editor: Antonio M. Esquinas
ISBN: 979-8-89530-264-4
© 2025 Nova Science Publishers, Inc.

Abbreviations

ATS	American Thoracic Society
CNS	Central nervous system
COPD	Chronic obstructive pulmonary disease
CRP	C-reactive protein
ERS	European Respiratory Society
FEV_1/FVC	The ratio of the forced expiratory volume in one second to the forced vital capacity
FVC	Forced vital capacity
FEV_1	Forced expiratory volume in one second
HFCWC	High-frequency chest wall compression
HFCWO	High-frequency chest wall oscillation
IL-6	Interleukin 6
LVEDP	Left ventricular end diastolic pressure
MV	Mechanical ventilation
NMBAs	Neuromuscular blocking agents
$PaCO_2$	Partial pressure of carbon dioxide in arteries
PaO_2	Partial pressure of oxygen in arteries
PEF	Peak expiratory flow
PR	Pulmonary rehabilitation
RF	Respiratory failure
SaO_2	Arterial oxygen saturation
SBT	Spontaneous breathing trial
VC	Vital capacity
WBC	White blood count
WOB	Work of breathing.

Pathophysiology of Ventilator Dependence

Mechanical ventilation (MV) becomes necessary when patients experience inadequate gas exchange or ventilatory capabilities in the respiratory system. This failure may stem by the lungs or by other organs including the cardiovascular system and central nervous system (CNS). This support may even occur due to the use of some medications such as anesthetic or neuromuscular blocking agents (NMBAs). However, not every instance requiring support defines ventilator dependence. Ventilator dependence refers to patients who have been under MV for more than 24 hours or who have failed attempts to be liberated from MV [1]. Clinicians typically identify reversible causes underlying ventilator dependence by examining the underlying pathophysiology. Often this pathophysiological outcome stems from the imbalance between capacity of respiratory muscles to function spontaneously and the demands placed on them after liberation from MV [2, 3].

Neurologic Factors

The respiratory center, located in the medulla oblongata and pons within the brainstem, acts as the controller responsible for generating the depth, rate, rhythm, and pattern of breathing. It receives feed-back from mechanoreceptors, chemoreceptors, and cortical sensors. Any disruption in feed-back mechanism or transmission of nerve impulses may predispose to respiratory failure. This failure may originate from central drive (e.g., coma, central apnea, cerebrovascular disease), peripheral nerves (e.g., phrenic nerve injury, iatrogenic phrenic nerve palsy), or metabolic factors (e.g., electrolyte disturbance) [1, 4].

Cardiovascular Factors

Although it presents as a respiratory mechanics issue, ventilator dependence can also be influenced by responses and changes in the cardiovascular system in patients under MV. Conditions like ischemia and heart failure may lead to ventilator dependence, and liberation attempts from the ventilator may also cause ischemia and heart failure. Increased metabolic load during spontaneous breathing, diaphragm contractions increasing venous return, and increases in left ventricular afterload caused by negative pleural pressure swings have been explained as cardiopulmonary interactions. Cardiopulmonary interactions occurring during liberation attempts from MV are defined as "weaning-induced cardiac dysfunction." This condition leads to decreased intrathoracic pressure, arterial oxygen saturation (SaO_2), and arterial partial pressure of oxygen (PaO_2), as well as increased work of breathing (WOB), arterial partial pressure of carbon dioxide ($PaCO_2$), and adrenergic tone. This can initiate an adverse cycle resulting in cardiogenic pulmonary edema and acute increase in left ventricular end diastolic pressure (LVEDP) [5, 6].

Metabolic Factors

Electrolyte and hormonal imbalances affect respiratory muscle function or WOB. Phosphate and magnesium deficiencies, bicarbonate excretion, and hypothyroidism impair normal ventilatory drive. Consequently, decreased SaO_2 and PaO_2 and increased $PaCO_2$ occur. This situation is most dramatically observed during systemic inflammatory diseases such as sepsis [1, 2].

Psychological Factors

Depression, sleep disturbances, anxiety, thanatophobia, delirium may constitute the majority of the non-respiratory factors causing ventilatory dependence. On the other hand, cognitive dysfunction, and dysregulation of circadian rhythm negatively contribute to the patient's psychological well-being [7].

Nutritional Factors

Nutrition is critical for patients under MV. During liberation, ventilator dependence may occur due to malnutrition, indicating a poor prognosis. The patient's energy needs must be calculated by indirect calorimetry or other valid measurement methods [2].

Respiratory Factors

The primary barriers to liberating from MV often involve the imbalance between the spontaneous load capacity of respiratory muscles and the demands faced after liberation from MV. Numerous studies in the literature attribute it to respiratory muscle weakness in mechanically ventilated patients. Pathophysiological sources of this weakness include atrophy or remodeling due to immobility, injury from overuse, neuropathy or myopathy associated with clinical condition, and myopathy resulting from polypharmacy. Conditions affecting the airway, such as asthma, chronic obstructive pulmonary disease (COPD), endotracheal intubation, tracheomalacia, tracheal stenosis can lead to various negative outcomes [2]. All these factors disrupt respiratory mechanics, thereby disrupting the balance between the spontaneous load production of the respiratory muscles and the load required liberation from MV. The specific evaluation challenges and lack of standardized methods in the literature have hindered clear demonstration of relationship between liberation from MV and ventilator dependence [1, 8].

Weaning

Discontinuation, withdrawal, or liberation from MV has been a hot topic among critical and respiratory care specialists since the polio pandemic in Copenhagen [9]. Although managing this process is a crucial clinical challenge, it demands specialized expertise. Patients may receive MV support based on the clinical condition of their diseases. As these conditions improve and stabilize, initiating the process of liberation from MV becomes a clinical task. This process, known as weaning, encompasses all interventions aimed at transitioning a patient from MV to spontaneous breathing. In summary, weaning is the journey from being under MV to achieving liberation from MV [2, 10].

Weaning involves a systemic approach for liberation from MV as soon as possible. This process is categorized into three types: simple, difficult, and prolonged [2]. Classification is based on objective evaluations during the spontaneous breathing trial (SBT) and SBT success in the prescribed period. Simple weaning is defined by successful evaluations within three SBTs and an average period of seven days. Since this process is linked to varying rates of incidence and mortality, it is crucial for clinicians to prioritize precautions. These include early interventions like early mobilization and SBT, as well as family support, psychological support, analgesia and sedation management, adequate and regular sleep [1].

High-Frequency Chest Wall Oscillation

High-frequency chest wall oscillation (HFCWO) involves a rigid shell or cuirass placed on the chest connected to a compressor that applies both positive and negative pressure to the chest wall [11]. In contrast, high-frequency chest wall compression (HFCWC) is a mechanical method that uses only positive pressure, applied via a vibrating vest [12]. Although these devices differ in engineering and technology, both methods are referred to as HFCWO in this chapter due to the lack of terminological standardization and their interchangeable use. This acceptance eliminates the distinction between compressor and material used. Thus, the definition in this chapter is: *"HFCWO is a mechanical method that causes inspiratory and expiratory flow oscillations by applying positive and negative, or only positive pressure to the chest wall."* The available HFCWO (only Hayek RTX Respirator) and HFCWC devices are listed in Figure 1.

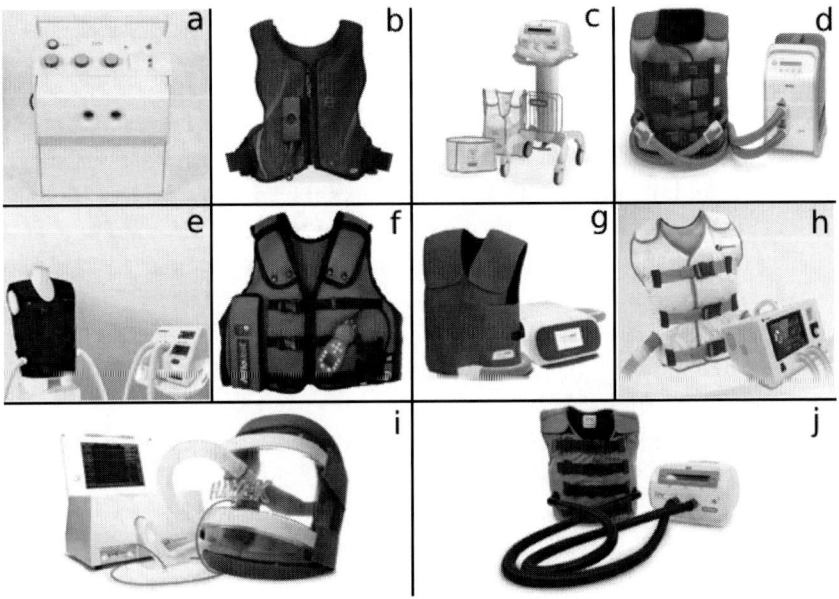

Figure 1. Different available HFCWO devices (with permissions).
a: ABI Vest Airway Clearance System (American Biosystems, St. Paul, MN USA); b: Monarch™ Airway Clearance System (Hill-Rom, Singapore, SG); c: The Vest® System Model 205 (Hill-Rom, Singapore, SG); d: The InCourage System (RespirTech, Lakeville, MN USA); e: CAREWAY (Korust Co., Gyeonggi-do, South Korea); f: AffloVest® (Tactile Medical, Minneapolis, MN USA); g: The SmartVest Airway Clearance System (Electromed, New Prague, MN USA); h: PneuVest (Lifotronic, Shenzhen, China); i: Hayek RTX Pespirator (Hayek Industries, London, United Kingdom); j: The Vest® System Model 105 (Hill-Rom, Singapore, SG).

High-frequency chest wall oscillation is an airway clearance therapy that stacks mini coughs into one spontaneous rapid exhalation. This method gained importance after King et al. reported 1983 study conducted on dogs that a 340% increase in tracheal mucus transport rate was observed. Although positive effects on forced vital capacity (FVC) and forced expiratory volume in one second (FEV_1) have been reported in several studies, its effects on airway clearance and respiratory function remain unclear. According to the clinical practice guidelines of the American College of Chest Physicians, this therapy is reported to have a low level of evidence and conflicting benefits for patients with cystic fibrosis [13].

High-Frequency Chest Wall Oscillation in Weaning

Liberation from MV may become difficult or unfeasible for various reasons. Prolonged immobility in endotracheally intubated patients can contribute to prolonged weaning times and reduced expectoration function. Impaired airway clearance due to factors such as pneumonia, MV, artificial airway can decrease SpO_2 and $PaCO_2$, worsen ventilation-perfusion matching and lead to atelectasis or lobar collapse [14]. Although the potential benefits of HFCWO for patients on prolonged MV are unknown, it represents a new technology that can be used for airway clearance.

A randomized controlled trial by Huang et al. on the elderly patients indicated that HFCWO could be safely applied after extubation altering physiological parameters such as blood pressure, heart rate, respiratory rate and SpO_2, potentially improving disease-related conditions [15]. Another study suggested that HFCWO after extubation in prolonged MV was more comfortable than conventional chest physiotherapy, but outcomes such as length of stay in hospital and intensive care unit, duration of MV, 30-day mortality, nosocomial pneumonia and lobar atelectasis were similar between both modalities [16]. A randomized controlled single-blinded study highlighted positive changes in peak inspiratory pressure and heart rate via HFCWO, without affecting ventilator settings or causing major changes in breathing patterns [14]. Additionally, a case report noted that combining HFCWO with conventional chest physiotherapy and mechanical insufflation-exsufflation in type 1 spinal muscular atrophy increased ventilator-free days, yet the potential benefits of HFCWO remained unproven [17].

The lack of conducted studies remains the primary barrier to publishing guidelines and recommendations. However, given the nature and potential benefits of HFCWO, its application in prolonged MV and weaning is crucial for future studies and clinical practices. Future studies that include cost effectiveness analysis in healthcare systems can further reinforce this importance.

Pulmonary Rehabilitation

Pulmonary rehabilitation (PR) is a core treatment approach that focuses on chronic respiratory patients, characterized as an individually tailored and multidisciplinary program. According to the ATS/ERS statement in 2006, pulmonary rehabilitation is described as "a comprehensive intervention based on thorough patient assessment followed by patient-tailored therapies that include, but are not limited to, exercise training, education, and behavior change, designed to improve the physical and psychological condition of people with chronic respiratory disease and to promote the long-term adherence to health-enhancing behaviors" [18].

Pulmonary rehabilitation is a well-established, clinically proven, and widely recognized therapeutic approach for improving the quality of life and functional capacity of patients with chronic respiratory diseases. The primary goals of PR include symptom control, particularly dyspnea, improvement in functional exercise performance, and reduction of symptoms related to depression and anxiety [19]. PR also aims to enhance health related quality of life and thereby reduce the frequency of hospitalizations. It has recently become the standard of care for various chronic respiratory diseases, encompassing conditions like bronchiectasis, interstitial lung disease, pulmonary fibrosis, post-tuberculosis lung disease, thoracic restriction, bronchiectasis, cystic fibrosis, asthma, pulmonary hypertension, pre and postoperative period of lung resection, volume reduction or transplantation and lung cancer [20].

The clinical relevance of PR may be "patient-centered," focusing on the individual respiratory condition, or "society-centered," considering disease epidemiology and societal costs. PR programs encompass several comprehensive, evidence-based components that go beyond exercise training to include patient assessment, education, and health enhancing behaviors [18, 21].

Impaired airway clearance is a common issue among patients with chronic respiratory diseases. In such cases, interventions like chest physiotherapy, manual airway clearance techniques, and mechanical airway clearance techniques are utilized. HFCWO can be employed within PR for patients having trouble with airway clearance. In the light of literature, HFCWO is well-tolerated and has been shown to significantly improve shortness of breath in adults hospitalized with acute asthma or COPD [22]. A study showed that using HFCWO for one year led to a significant decrease in all-cause hospital stays, oral and intravenous antibiotics usage, and radiology examinations in patients with bronchiectasis. Furthermore, there was a reduction in patient-specific hospitalizations, acute exacerbations, outpatient visits, and use of radiology and laboratory services [23].

The literature has shown that the use of HFCWO can improve symptoms such as sputum production, shortness of breath, and cough. It also enhances blood gas and pulmonary function parameters including PaO_2, $PaCO_2$, FVC, PEF, VC, FEV_1 and FEV_1/FVC. Cheng et al. reported positive improvements in inflammatory indicators such as WBC, CRP, and IL-6 [24].

Despite the current literature suggesting that HFCWO is effective and safe for patients with chronic respiratory diseases or in PR, studies are limited in terms of standardization, recommendations, and preparation guidelines. Therefore, new studies, recommendations and guidelines investigating the use of HFCWO in PR are needed.

Conclusion

High-frequency Chest Wall Oscillation, introduced in the early 1980s, still has limited applications today, and its underlying concept remains incompletely understood. There is an urgent need for industry and clinicians to establish a common terminology and accurately differentiate between the compressor and oscillator mechanisms used in HFCWO modalities, which are frequently misinterpreted. Therefore, it is crucial to emphasize that the literature recognizes two distinct modalities: high-frequency chest wall compression (HFCWC) and high-frequency chest wall oscillation (HFCWO).

HFCWO is primarily used in cystic fibrosis treatment. However, recent studies have increasingly investigated its application beyond this condition. With demonstrated efficacy in airway clearance and improving respiratory function, HFCWO has shown versatility across various medical conditions. Its potential for safe and effective integration into PR, leveraging its well-established physiological benefits, is promising. Additionally, in intensive care settings, HFCWO has shown promise in managing secretions and potentially reducing MV dependence. Consequently, comprehensive clinical studies are essential to fully explore HFWCO's potential in both PR and intensive care, particularly in reducing MV dependence.

Key Messages

1. HFCWO can potentially be used across various healthcare settings, however its safety, effectiveness, and cost-effectiveness remain unclear.
2. Given the promising benefits observed in a limited number of studies, HFCWO may be considered as an adjunct or standard applications during prolonged MV and weaning.
3. New studies, recommendations and guidelines are necessary to investigate the application of HFCWO in PR.
4. Standardizing terminology such as HFCWO and HFCWC in the literature is essential, considering their engineering and technological differences.

References

[1] MacIntyre NR, Cook DJ, Ely EW Jr, Epstein SK, Fink JB, Heffner JE, Hess D, Hubmayer RD, Scheinhorn DJ; American College of Chest Physicians; American Association for Respiratory Care; American College of Critical Care Medicine. Evidence-based guidelines for weaning and discontinuing ventilatory support: a collective task force facilitated by the American College of Chest Physicians; the American Association for Respiratory Care; and the American College of Critical Care Medicine. *Chest.* 2001 Dec;120(6 Suppl):375S-95S.

[2] Akella P, Voigt LP, Chawla S. To Wean or Not to Wean: A Practical Patient Focused Guide to Ventilator Weaning. *J Intensive Care Med.* 2022 Nov;37(11):1417-1425.

[3] Sandoval Moreno LM, Casas Quiroga IC, Wilches Luna EC, Garcia AF. Efficacy of respiratory muscle training in weaning of mechanical ventilation in patients with mechanical ventilation for 48 hours or more: a randomized controlled clinical trial. *Med Intensiva.* 2019;43(2):79–89.

[4] Doorduin J, Haans AJC, Hoeven J, Heunks L. Difficult weaning: principles and practice of a structured diagnostic approach. *Netherlands Journal of Critical Care.* 2013;17(4):11.

[5] Teboul JL. Weaning-induced cardiac dysfunction: where are we today? *Intensive Care Med.* 2014 Aug;40(8):1069-79.

[6] Routsi C, Stanopoulos I, Kokkoris S, Sideris A, Zakynthinos S. Weaning failure of cardiovascular origin: how to suspect, detect and treat-a review of the literature. *Ann Intensive Care.* 2019 Jan 9;9(1):6.

[7] Pandharipande PP, Girard TD, Jackson JC, Morandi A, Thompson JL, Pun BT, Brummel NE, Hughes CG, Vasilevskis EE, Shintani AK, Moons KG, Geevarghese SK, Canonico A, Hopkins RO, Bernard GR, Dittus RS, Ely EW; BRAIN-ICU Study

Investigators. Long-term cognitive impairment after critical illness. *N Engl J Med.* 2013 Oct 3;369(14):1306-16.

[8] Tobin MJ, Guenther SM, Perez W, Lodato RF, Mador MJ, Allen SJ, Dantzker DR. Konno-Mead analysis of ribcage-abdominal motion during successful and unsuccessful trials of weaning from mechanical ventilation. *Am Rev Respir Dis.* 1987 Jun;135(6):1320-8.

[9] Ibsen B. The anaesthetist's viewpoint on the treatment of respiratory complications in poliomyelitis during the epidemic in Copenhagen, 1952. *Proc R Soc Med.* 1954 Jan;47(1):72-4.

[10] Macintyre NR. Evidence-based assessments in the ventilator discontinuation process. *Respir Care.* 2012 Oct;57(10):1611-8.

[11] Chatburn RL. High-frequency assisted airway clearance. *Respir Care.* 2007 Sep; 52(9):1224-35; discussion 1235-7.

[12] Ntoumenopoulos G. High-frequency chest wall compressions: good for the patient? Good for the clinician? *Respir Care.* 2012 Feb;57(2):323-5.

[13] McCool FD, Rosen MJ. Nonpharmacologic airway clearance therapies: ACCP evidence-based clinical practice guidelines. *Chest.* 2006 Jan;129(1 Suppl):250S-259S.

[14] Chuang ML, Chou YL, Lee CY, Huang SF. Instantaneous responses to high-frequency chest wall oscillation in patients with acute pneumonic respiratory failure receiving mechanical ventilation: A randomized controlled study. *Medicine* (Baltimore). 2017 Mar;96(9):e5912.

[15] Huang WC, Wu PC, Chen CJ, Cheng YH, Shih SJ, Chen HC, Wu CL. High-frequency chest wall oscillation in prolonged mechanical ventilation patients: a randomized controlled trial. *Clin Respir J.* 2016 May;10(3):272-81.

[16] Clinkscale D, Spihlman K, Watts P, Rosenbluth D, Kollef MH. A randomized trial of conventional chest physical therapy versus high-frequency chest wall compressions in intubated and non-intubated adults. *Respir Care.* 2012 Feb;57(2): 221-8.

[17] Keating JM, Collins N, Bush A, Chatwin M. High-frequency chest-wall oscillation in a noninvasive-ventilation-dependent patient with type 1 spinal muscular atrophy. *Respir Care.* 2011 Nov;56(11):1840-3.

[18] Spruit MA, Singh SJ, Garvey C, ZuWallack R, Nici L, Rochester C, Hill K, Holland AE, Lareau SC, Man WD, Pitta F, Sewell L, Raskin J, Bourbeau J, Crouch R, Franssen FM, Casaburi R, Vercoulen JH, Vogiatzis I, Gosselink R, Clini EM, Effing TW, Maltais F, van der Palen J, Troosters T, Janssen DJ, Collins E, Garcia-Aymerich J, Brooks D, Fahy BF, Puhan MA, Hoogendoorn M, Garrod R, Schols AM, Carlin B, Benzo R, Meek P, Morgan M, Rutten-van Mölken MP, Ries AL, Make B, Goldstein RS, Dowson CA, Brozek JL, Donner CF, Wouters EF; ATS/ERS Task Force on Pulmonary Rehabilitation. An official American Thoracic Society/European Respiratory Society statement: key concepts and advances in pulmonary rehabilitation. *Am J Respir Crit Care Med.* 2013 Oct 15;188(8):e13-64.

[19] Gordon CS, Waller JW, Cook RM, Cavalera SL, Lim WT, Osadnik CR. Effect of Pulmonary Rehabilitation on Symptoms of Anxiety and Depression in COPD. *Chest.* 2019 Jul;156(1):80–91.

[20] Cesario A, Ferri L, Galetta D, Pasqua F, Bonassi S, Clini E, et al. Post-operative respiratory rehabilitation after lung resection for non-small cell lung cancer. *Lung Cancer*. 2007 Aug;57(2):175–80.

[21] Panagiotou M, Polychronopoulos V, Strange C. Respiratory and lower limb muscle function in interstitial lung disease. *Chron Respir Dis*. 2016 May;13(2):162–72.

[22] Mahajan AK, Diette GB, Hatipoğlu U, Bilderback A, Ridge A, Harris VW, Dalapathi V, Badlani S, Lewis S, Charbeneau JT, Naureckas ET, Krishnan JA. High-frequency chest wall oscillation for asthma and chronic obstructive pulmonary disease exacerbations: a randomized sham-controlled clinical trial. *Respir Res*. 2011 Sep 10;12(1):120.

[23] Martha E. Camacho Urribarri, Brian C. Becker, Angela C. Murray, Impact of High-Frequency Chest Wall Oscillation on Health Care Resource Use and Economic Outcomes in Adult Patients With Non-Cystic Fibrosis Bronchiectasis in the United States: A Pre-Post Cohort Analysis, *CHEST Pulmonary*, 2023 Aug 18.

[24] Cheng G, Wu J, Hu Z, Xiao Y, Zeng B, Zhou Y. Effects of High-Frequency Chest Wall Oscillation Expectoration System on Pulmonary Rehabilitation and Cortisol Function in Patients with Severe AECOPD. *Dis Markers*. 2022 Jul 22;2022: 3380048.

Chapter 11

High-Frequency Chest Wall Oscillation in Extubation Respiratory Failure

Inês Martinho Santos Jorge[*], MD
Physical and Rehabilitation Medicine, Unidade Local de Saúde do Alto Minho, Viana do Castelo, Portugal

Abstract

Extubation failure is common in intensive care units (ICUs). It corresponds to an inability to maintain spontaneous breathing after artificial airway removal (an endotracheal tube or tracheostomy tube) and need for reintubation within 24-72 hours or up to 7 days.

Substantial literature exists about weaning predictors and outcomes. Most of them being inaccurate in predicting extubation outcomes. To predict extubation failure is essential. Both delayed and failed extubation have severe consequences, such as prolonged ventilation, a need for tracheostomy, increased time of stay in the ICU and hospital, increased cost of treatment, and greater risk of morbidity and mortality.

The risk of extubation failure is increased in patients with advanced age, high severity of illness at ICU admission, preexisting chronic respiratory and cardiovascular disorders.

Parameters used to predict extubation failure can be categorized into assessing respiratory mechanics, airway patency and protection and cardiovascular reserve. An effective cough, a small amount of bronchial secretions and good alertness are necessary for a successful extubation. Multidisciplinary teams (intensivists, pulmonologists, physiatrists) combined with the implementation of ventilatory weaning protocols favor successful weaning and lower reintubation rates.

---

[*] Corresponding Author's Email: inessantosjorge@gmail.com.

In: High-frequency Chest Wall Oscillation Therapy in Critical Ill Patients
Editor: Antonio M. Esquinas
ISBN: 979-8-89530-264-4
© 2025 Nova Science Publishers, Inc.

Keywords: extubation, postextubation respiratory failure, weaning, predictors, intensive care unit

Introduction

Liberation from mechanical ventilation is a three-step process that involves readiness testing, weaning, and extubation [1]. In this chapter we highlight the last one.

Extubation refers to removal of the endotracheal tube and it is the third and last step in liberating a patient from mechanical ventilation. It is performed when the patient is successful at weaning and both airway patency and airway protection measures are in place. Extubation should not be performed until it has been determined that the patient's medical condition is stable, the airway is patent, and any potential difficulties in reintubation have been identified. In general, most patients in the intensive care unit (ICU) should not be extubated unless a successful weaning trial has been passed [1]. Exceptions include postoperative patients who are recovered for short periods in the ICU (e.g., 24 hours) and patients undergoing terminal extubation. One study showed a decrease rate of reintubation at 48 hours when patients were rested back on the ventilator for an hour before extubation after the completion of a spontaneous breathing trial.

For extubation, patients should have normal oxygenation and adequate weaning parameters, such as a rapid and superficial respiratory rate below 105 breaths/minute/liter. An upper airway anatomy assessment is important for the danger of significant laryngeal edema.

However, some patients fail ventilatory extubation. Failed extubation is defined as the need for reinstitution of ventilatory support within 24 to 72 hours of planned endotracheal tube removal, this occurs in 2 to 25% of extubated patients [1]. It is associated with extremely poor outcomes, including high mortality rates of 25 to 50% [2].

Definition

Postextubation respiratory failure (within 72 hours) is defined as the presence and persistence of respiratory acidosis (pH <7.35), hypercapnia (PaCO2 >45 mmHg), SPO2 less than 90% or PaO2 less than 60 mmHg on FiO2 higher than

0.4, respiratory rate greater than 35, decreased level of consciousness, agitation and clinical signs suggesting respiratory muscle fatigue and increased work of breathing [3].

Pathophysiology

The pathophysiologic causes of extubation failure include an imbalance between respiratory muscle capacity and work of breathing, upper airway obstruction, excess respiratory secretions, inadequate cough, encephalopathy, and cardiac dysfunction. Compared with patients who tolerate extubation, those who require reintubation have a higher incidence of hospital mortality, increased length of ICU and hospital stay, prolonged duration of mechanical ventilation, higher hospital costs, and an increased need for tracheostomy [1]. Given the lack of proven treatments for extubation failure, clinicians must be aware of the factors that predict extubation outcome to improve clinical decision making [1].

Extubation Failure

Patients at high risk for extubation failure frequently have significant comorbidity, prolonged intubation periods and poor weaning trials. Some patients have significant respiratory impairment prior to hospitalization and in these cases, it may be quite difficult to determine whether or not they are at their baseline [2]. Reintubation of these patients increases morbidity and mortality which has exceeded 40% in some studies.

High risk factors for reintubation included older age (greater than 65 y.o.), Acute Physiology and Chronic Health Evaluation II (APACHE II) score greater than 12, body mass index greater than 30 kg/m^2, inadequate secretions management, difficult or prolonged weaning, more than one comorbidity, heart failure as an indication for mechanical ventilation, moderate to severe chronic obstructive pulmonary disease (COPD), airway patency problems, and prolonged mechanical ventilation or hypercapnia on finishing the spontaneous breathing trial [3, 4].

There is some evidence that extubation failure can directly worsen patient outcomes independently of underlying illness severity. Two preventive measures may prove beneficial, although their exact role needs confirmation:

one is noninvasive ventilation after extubation in high-risk or hypercapnic patients, and the other is steroid administration several hours before extubation. These measures might help to prevent postextubation respiratory distress in selected patient subgroups [2].

Diaphragm Evaluation

Diaphragm is the main respiratory muscle which plays a crucial role in ventilation. Trans-diaphragmatic pressure measurement is considered to be the gold standard for diaphragm dysfunction diagnoses. Ultrasound is a noninvasive exam which allows diaphragm visualization and its variation during respiratory cycles. Two main parameters for evaluating diaphragmatic function are diaphragmatic excursion and diaphragmatic thickening.

Diaphragmatic excursion is measured with a 3-5MHz probe on the midclavicular line, below the rib margin and oriented dorsally to visualize excursion of the diaphragm dome, using the liver (or spleen, on the left side) as an acoustic window. An excursion less than 10 mm for hemidiaphragm is associated to longer weaning times and greater frequency of reintubation. So, diaphragmatic excursion can predict weaning failure but the index respiratory frequency/diaphragmatic excursion in mm has shown better results to predict [4].

Diaphragmatic thickening during inspiration is measured with a 10MHz probe over the ninth intercostal space, in the diaphragm positioning zone. We can measure the maximum (at inspiration end) and the minimum (at expiration end) diaphragmatic thickness, with calculation of *thickening fraction* (thickness at inspiration end/thickness expiration end). A thickening fraction of 30-36% is associated with weaning success. In patients ventilated in pressure support mode, diaphragmatic thickening is correlated to invasive parameters of diaphragmatic pressure, being a reliable indicator of respiratory effort. In contrast, excursion is not correlated to respiratory effort, and only reflects passive displacement of the diaphragmatic due to the pressure generated by the ventilator. It therefore should only be used in those patients in which spontaneous breathing trial (SBT) is performed in T-tube [5].

In recent years, diaphragmatic ultrasound has been used for this purpose. Patients on MV may have a multifactorial deterioration of diaphragmatic function can lead to weaning failure and prolongation of invasive mechanical ventilation; therefore, assessing diaphragmatic function could help predict the patient's ability to maintain spontaneous breathing over times. However, this is a technique that requires experience.

Prevention

To prevent extubation failure, the last clinical practice guidelines on liberation from mechanical ventilation suggest conducting the initial SBT with inspiratory pressure augmentation and recommend preventive NIV for patients at high risk for extubation failure. The wide range of respiratory support, from automatic tube compensation to pressure support up to 10 cm H_2O, generates a heterogeneous response that makes predicting the outcome difficult, leading to important clinical consequences. The results of a study showed that 1-hour reconnection to mechanical ventilation after a tolerated SBT significantly reduced the reintubation rate in a population of patients who underwent SBT mostly by T-tube [5]. This result suggests that highly demanding SBT can contribute to extubation failure.

Positive end-expiratory pressure (PEEP) also generates controversy; the studies analyzed used a PEEP level ranging from 0 to 5 cm H2O, and protocols for preventive therapy after extubation always include PEEP.

The main result of this study is that inspiratory pressure augmentation significantly increased the proportion of patients successfully extubated when a preventive therapy was planned, reinforcing the idea that inspiratory pressure augmentation will probably hasten the extubation in these patients [6].

Note: Although SBT is an appropriate way to prepare the patient for extubation, even after successful SBT, failure rates and subsequent reintubation can exceed 20% in the highest-risk patients.

Management

Postextubation management usually includes conventional oxygenation with facemasks. Alternative approaches use noninvasive ventilation and high flow nasal cannula oxygenation. High flow nasal oxygen delivery has been used especially for oxygen supplementation in patients with acute hypoxemic respiratory failure. Hernández et al. recently reported a randomized controlled trial which have shown that high-flow nasal cannula (HFNC) oxygen therapy was noninferior to noninvasive ventilation (NIV) for preventing reintubation in a heterogeneous population at high-risk for extubation failure. In addition, adverse events were less frequent in the high flow nasal cannula group. However, outcomes might differ in certain subgroups of patients [7]. Among adult critically ill patients at very high-risk for extubation failure, NIV with active humidification was superior to HFNC for preventing reintubation [7].

Cough augmentation techniques, such as lung volume recruitment or manually and mechanically assisted cough, are important to prevent and manage respiratory complications associated with chronic conditions, particularly neuromuscular disease, and may improve short- and long-term outcomes for people with acute respiratory failure [8].

Conclusion

The process of weaning from mechanical ventilation remains one of the most critical challenges in patients undergoing mechanical ventilation in the ICU. The multidisciplinary team must study the optimal time for weaning from the mechanical ventilation. Several measurements have been used to predict the success of weaning from mechanical ventilation; however, their efficacy varies in different studies. So, clinical medical assessment must be sovereign. The patient must be approached as a whole and not just the values given by the ventilator must be taken into consideration. HFCWO could be a rational therapy to improve and control airway secretions during weaning from mechanical ventilation and prevent postextubation respiratory failure.

Key Messages

1. Weaning from mechanical ventilation is a critical issue in Critical Care
2. A multidisciplinary approach and use of airway clearance secretions management is essential in prevention and treatment respiratory failure.
3. Early use of HFCWO in mechanical ventilated patients is essential to prevent postextubation respiratory failure associated with airway secretions.

References

[1] Rothaar RC, Epstein SK. Extubation failure: magnitude of the problem, impact on outcomes, and prevention. *Curr Opin Crit Care* 2003 Feb;9(1):59-66. doi: 10.1097/00075198-200302000-00011.

[2] Thille AW, Richard JC, Brochard L. The decision to extubate in the intensive care unit. *Am J Respir Crit Care Med* 2013 Jun 15;187(12):1294-302. doi: 10.1164/rccm.201208-1523CI.

[3] Hernández G, et al. Effect of postextubation noninvasive ventilation with active humidification vs high-flow nasal cannula on reintubation in patients at very high risk for extubation failure: a randomized trial. *Intensive Care Med* 2022 Dec;48(12):1751-1759. doi: 10.1007/s00134-022-06919-3. Epub 2022 Nov 18. Erratum in: Intensive Care Med. 2023 Mar;49(3):385.

[4] Nugent K. Postextubation management of patients at high risk for reintubation. *J Thorac Dis.* 2016 Dec;8(12): E1679-E1682. doi: 10.21037/jtd.2016.12.96.

[5] Zapata L, Blancas R, Conejo-Márquez I, García-de-Acilu M. Role of ultrasound in acute respiratory failure and in the weaning of mechanical ventilation. *Med Intensiva (Engl Ed)* 2023 Sep;47(9):529-542. doi: 10.1016/j.medine.2023.03.018.

[6] Hernandez G, Roca O. Redefining "Minimal Ventilator Settings": Should We Customize the Spontaneous Breathing Trial in the Era of Prevention of Extubation Failure? *Chest* 2020 Oct;158(4):1314-1316. doi: 10.1016/j.chest.2020.05.578.

[7] Jha AK. Postextubation ventilation strategy in preventing reintubation in patients at very high risk for extubation failure. *Intensive Care Med* 2023 Mar;49(3):374-375.

[8] Rose L, Adhikari NK, Leasa D, Fergusson DA, McKim D. Cough augmentation techniques for extubation or weaning critically ill patients from mechanical ventilation. *Cochrane Database Syst Rev* 2017 Jan 11;1(1):CD011833. doi: 10.1002/14651858.CD011833.pub2.

Chapter 12

High-Frequency Chest Wall Oscillation in Chronic Obstructive Pulmonary Disorder

Salvatore Notaro[*]
Vincezo Capaldo
Andrea Imparato
and Eugenio Piscitelli
Department of Critical Care, Intensive Care Units And ECMO, Monaldi-Colli Hospital, Naples, Italy

Abstract

COPD is a disease characterized by persistent respiratory symptoms and airflow limitation due to airway and/or alveolar abnormalities. It is usually caused by significant exposure to noxious particles or gases and is the third most common cause of death globally. For the diagnosis, the presence of three features: spirometric alterations, clinical symptoms, and exposure to noxious stimuli is necessary. A characteristic is the production of mucus, which increases during exacerbations accompanied by infection, atelectasis, and respiratory difficulties. Treatment includes both drug-based and non-drug-based approaches in both stable and exacerbation phases. Drug-based therapy involves using LAMA, LABA, and ICS either individually or in combination depending on the type. It also involves oxygen therapy with various respiratory supports based on the severity of the condition. Non-drug-based therapy includes traditional physiotherapy as well as modern techniques. High-Frequency Chest Wall Oscillation (HFCWO) is an effective modern respiratory physiotherapy technique. It involves using a wearable vest connected to a pressure

---

[*] Corresponding Author's Email: notaro@hotmail.it.

In: High-frequency Chest Wall Oscillation Therapy in Critical Ill Patients
Editor: Antonio M. Esquinas
ISBN: 979-8-89530-264-4
© 2025 Nova Science Publishers, Inc.

generator that applies high-frequency compressions to the chest wall. This action helps release mucus from the peripheral airways, mimicking the cough mechanism and promoting mucus clearance. Numerous clinical studies have demonstrated the effectiveness of this technique, showing improvements in respiratory mechanics, gas exchange, and reduced respiratory effort. Additionally, it is highly suitable for home use and has been shown to improve quality of life. Therefore, it can be concluded that HFCWO is a safe and effective technique compared to traditional physiotherapy.

Keywords: chronic obstructive pulmonary disease, mucociliary clearance, physiotherapy, airway secretions devices, HFCWO

Introduction

Chronic Obstructive Pulmonary Disease (COPD) is a condition marked by ongoing respiratory symptoms and restricted airflow, resulting from airway and/or alveolar irregularities, usually as a result of significant exposure to harmful particles or gases. It is the third leading cause of death worldwide [1]. Diagnosis requires the presence of three specific changes in spirometry, along with clinical symptoms and exposure to noxious stimuli. One of the characteristics of COPD is the production of mucus, which increases during exacerbations accompanied by infection, atelectasis, and respiratory difficulties. Treatment for COPD includes both pharmacological and non-pharmacological approaches, both during stable periods and exacerbations. Oxygen therapy with various respiratory supports is used depending on the severity of the condition. Non-pharmacological therapy includes traditional physiotherapy as well as modern techniques. One effective modern technique is High-frequency Chest Wall Oscillation (HFCWO) [2]. This involves the use of a wearable vest connected to a pressure generator that applies high-frequency compressions to the chest wall. This helps release mucus from the peripheral airways, simulates the cough mechanism, and aids in mucociliary clearance. Clinical studies have shown that HFCWO is effective and safe compared to traditional physiotherapy. HFCWO is considered a modern and reliable treatment option for COPD patients. This chapter aims to discuss HFCWO as a technique for managing airway secretions in COPD patients.

Definition

Chronic obstructive pulmonary disease (COPD) is a common, preventable, and treatable condition characterized by persistent respiratory symptoms and airflow limitation. This is usually caused by significant exposure to harmful particles or gases [1, 2]. The Global Initiative for Chronic Obstructive Lung Disease (GOLD) was established in 1998 by the National Heart, Lung, and Blood Institute to address COPD [2]. Since 2001, GOLD periodically publishes a consensus report outlining a global strategy for the Diagnosis, Management, and Prevention of COPD. This report was developed by an international panel of health professionals from various fields. The objectives of the GOLD initiative are to improve the diagnosis and management of COPD worldwide. COPD affects approximately 1 in 10 adults globally and is one of the leading causes of death. In 2019, it claimed 3.22 million lives, with a 17.5% increase in deaths from 2007 to 2017 [3]. The highest burden of mortality from COPD is observed in several regions, including Latin America, sub-Saharan Africa, India, China, and Southeast Asia. According to the Global Burden of Disease study, in 2015, COPD affected 104.7 million men and 69.7 million women globally, with a 44.2% increase in prevalence from 1990 to 2015 [4-6]. The treatment of COPD involves both pharmacological and non-pharmacological approaches, with non-pharmacological options including traditional and modern physiotherapy treatments.

Diagnosis

As per GOLD guidelines, the diagnosis of COPD necessitates the presence of three features: 1) a post-bronchodilator forced expiratory volume in 1 second (FEV_1)/forced vital capacity (FVC) ratio of less than 0.70, which confirms the existence of persistent airflow limitation, 2) appropriate symptoms including dyspnea, chronic cough, sputum production, or wheezing, and 3) significant exposures to noxious stimuli such as a history of smoking cigarettes or other environmental exposures [7].

Pharmacological and Non-Pharmacological Management

Pharmacological Management

Pharmacological therapy for chronic obstructive pulmonary disease (COPD) includes the use of LAMA, LABA, ICS either individually or in combination, depending on the specific type of COPD. According to the 2018 GOLD document, there is new supporting evidence for the use of triple therapy with LABA/LAMA/ICS [8]. Long-term oxygen therapy is recommended for COPD patients with a resting oxygen saturation (SaO2) of 88% or less, or arterial oxygen partial pressure of 55 mm Hg or less. It is also suggested for patients with coexisting conditions such as pulmonary hypertension, congestive heart failure, or polycythemia (hematocrit > 55%), at an arterial oxygen partial pressure between 55 and 60mm Hg, or an SaO2 of 88% to 93%. Once prescribed, it is recommended to aim for ana SaO2 of greater than or equal to 90%, and to periodically reassess the need for and the effectiveness of the prescription. The use of noninvasive ventilation is recommended for the treatment of patients with exacerbating hypercapnic respiratory failure [9-10]. For patients with advanced emphysema or large bullae, the guidelines suggest considering bullectomy, lung volume reduction, or lung transplantation [11-12].

Exacerbations of COPD

The GOLD 2023 proposes a more specific definition of ECOPD as an event characterized by increased dyspnea and/or cough and sputum that worsens in less than 14 days. This may be accompanied by tachypnea and/or tachycardia and is often associated with increased local and systemic inflammation caused by infection, pollution, or other insults to the airways [13]. COPD exacerbations not only bring financial burdens, increased healthcare utilization, and disruptiveness but also pose risks of death, iatrogenic complications, setbacks to quality of life, and faster decline of lung function [14-15]. The management of exacerbations, as well as the GOLD guidelines, has not substantially changed. A mild exacerbation requires a temporary step-up in short-acting bronchodilators alone, while a moderate exacerbation requires systemic corticosteroids or antibiotics, or both. A severe exacerbation is defined by the treatment received at the emergency department or hospital.

It is recommended to use systemic corticosteroids at a modest dose (40 mg) and for a short course (5-7 days). Successful COPD action plans often include dual prescriptions for oral corticosteroids and antibiotics. A 5- to 7-day antibiotic course is recommended for exacerbations with increased sputum purulence or the need for mechanical ventilation (invasive or noninvasive). Antibiotic therapy reduces mortality for COPD exacerbations that require intensive care and reduces treatment failure in the inpatient setting, with more modest benefits in the outpatient setting. Instead of advocating for a specific antibiotic, the selection is based on local resistance patterns and a preference for oral versus intravenous route of administration [16]. Oxygen therapy is recommended to achieve an oxygen saturation of 88% to 92%. Over-oxygenation is associated with increased hypercapnia and mortality. Noninvasive positive pressure ventilation (NIPPV) is the first-line therapy for hypercapnic respiratory failure ($PCO_2 > 45$ mm Hg and arterial pH 7.35). Contraindications to NIPPV include emesis, inability to protect the airway, and the need for urgent intubation. Proper usage of NIPPV successfully improves oxygenation, pH, and work of breathing, leading to significant decreases in mortality and intubation rates [17]. High flow oxygen by nasal cannula (HFNC) is recommended for the treatment of ECOPD with hypoxemic respiratory failure.

Non-Pharmacological Management

Non-pharmacological treatment is a key part of the appropriate management of COPD and should always be considered in combination with pharmacologic treatment. It includes one or more of the following: education and supported self-management, smoking cessation, vaccination, and physical activity.

Pulmonary Rehabilitation

The guidelines recommend comprehensive pulmonary rehabilitation and discuss its various components. During exacerbation, the amount and viscosity of secretions increase, and mucus clearance is impaired, resulting in an increase in respiratory infections similar to bronchiectasis and cystic fibrosis. This alteration of the mucociliary mechanism contributes to the impairment of mucociliary clearance, promoting mucus-stasis and the increased retention of bronchial secretions as a result of mucociliary dysfunction, reduced cough function, and weakness of the inspiratory and expiratory muscles. This ultimately obstructs the airways, leading to ventilation/perfusion mismatch, hypoxemia, and respiratory fatigue. The accumulation of mucus in small and basilar airways causes atelectasis and increases the risk of developing pneumonia, potentially leading to acute respiratory failure requiring intensive care and increasing mortality. Maintenance of airway secretion clearance, or airway hygiene, is important for preserving airway patency. Removing mucus clearance is of fundamental importance in such cases, as mucus drainage increases oxygenation, improves pulmonary functions and exercise capacity, and decreases the frequency of respiratory infections [18].

Traditional pulmonary physiotherapy, including percussion, vibration, cough maneuvers, forced expiration techniques, postural drainage, and shaking, is used to mobilize mucus in patients with respiratory diseases. Modern pulmonary physiotherapy techniques, such as Intrapulmonary percussive devices (IPV-1S Universal Percussionator, Percussionaire, Sandpoint, Idaho; PercussiveNeb, Vortran Medical Technology, Sacramento, California; IMP2, Breas Medical, Mölnlycke, Sweden), various vest devices (Hill-Rom the Vest Airway Clearance System, Hill-Rom, St Paul, Minnesota; SmartVest, Electromed, New Prague, Minnesota; inCourage, RespirTech, St Paul, Minnesota), and active devices such as the Hayek oscillator, are used to increase mucus clearance in patients with respiratory diseases, particularly cystic fibrosis. These assisted airways cleaning techniques (ACT) create both positive and negative trans-respiratory pressure alterations via high-frequency, leading to low-volume oscillations in the airways and the mobilization of secretions. In traditional manual therapies, patients need an assistant physiotherapist. However, with the modern physiotherapy approach, techniques that can be applied by the patients themselves have been used more frequently [19].

High-Frequency Chest Wall Oscillation

High-frequency chest wall oscillation is a modern physiotherapy technique that involves wearing a vest connected to an air generator. The device creates oscillations in the chest wall, providing external chest wall oscillation per second (Figure 1). The oscillations help improve the interaction between airflow and mucus, reducing the viscoelasticity of the secretions.

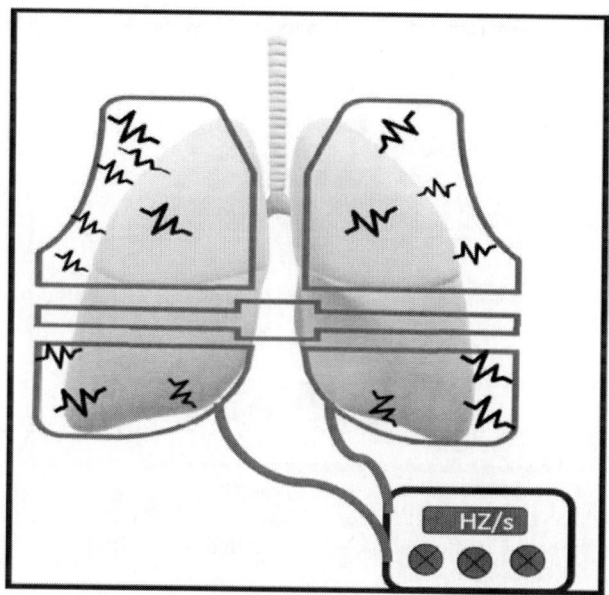

Figure 1. HFCWO vest and device. Wearable vest and air generator device that creates oscillations in the chest wall. Provides 20 Hz external chest wall oscillations per second. It is applied using an inflatable vest attached to a machine that vibrates at variable frequencies and intensities.

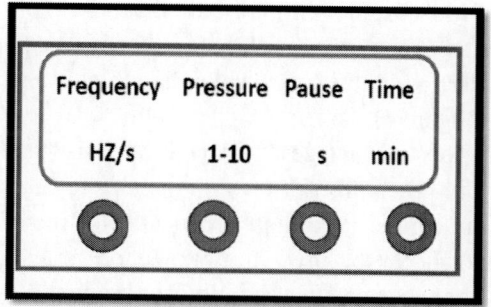

Figure 2. Device. Parameters to be set in some devices.

The vest is inflatable and attached to a device (Figure 2), which is a machine that produces vibrations at variable frequencies and intensities, adjusted by the operator to ensure the individual's comfort and compliance. Compression can be initiated using hands or feet, allowing the individual to apply it on their own.

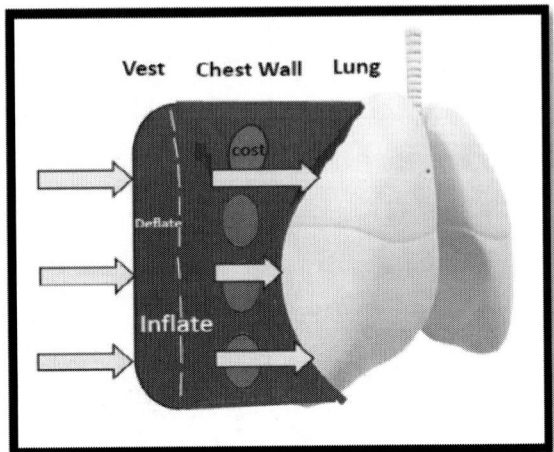

Figure 3. Vest on the chest wall. Effect of inflating and deflating the vest, the pressure generated (yellow arrow) is transmitted to the chest wall, from there to the lung parenchyma and bronchi.

The oscillations are generated by the device with a frequency of 5–25 Hz and transmitted through the chest wall to the entire bronchial tree (Figure 3). The pressure variable setting is 2–5 cm H2O to achieve a tight but comfortable fit based on individual patient tolerance The device has been shown to be as effective as conventional physiotherapy and is frequently preferred by patients due to its ease of use and suitability for individual use [20].

The air generator can vibrate at a high-frequency by compressing the chest wall, increasing airflow in the lungs and aiding the expulsion of mucus from bronchial walls (Figure 4).

One of the key advantages of the device is that it can be used simultaneously with a nebulizer. It is recommended to be used twice a day for 20-30 minutes but can be used more frequently for more severe symptoms (every 3-4 hours). It can be used in any position to avoid aspiration. It is commonly used for patients with cystic fibrosis, bronchiectasis, and other lung diseases, and can be used for a lifetime.

High-frequency chest wall oscillation is recommended for patients with cystic fibrosis, bronchiectasis, ciliary dyskinesia syndrome, lung cavity diseases, and muscular pulmonary dysfunction. It is also a good option for mentally retarded patients and those with neuromuscular diseases [21].

In 1985, King et al. first used a high-frequency chest wall oscillation (HFCWO) device on dogs. Studies in dogs showed that it increased tracheal mucus clearance compared to controls. Subsequent studies on humans confirmed that the device effectively clears tracheal mucus secretion [22]. The main mechanism of action involves increasing mucus secretion by generating expiratory flow higher than inspiratory flow, similar to normal coughing. This mechanism helps to clear bronchial secretions, mimicking tiny coughs.

The HFCWO device creates lung percussion to clean the peripheral bronchial tree, directing secretions toward the large airways and facilitating their removal. This device is mainly used for bronchiectasis and cystic fibrosis patients to reduce bronchial obstruction, improve expectoration, and enhance oxygenation. Studies in cystic fibrosis (CF) patients have indicated that HFCWO can significantly reduce healthcare costs and lung infection rates in CF [23]. Research on various patient groups has also demonstrated that HFCWO provides better mucus clearance and improved respiratory function compared to conventional chest physiotherapy. Additionally, studies have shown a decrease in mucus viscosity with HFCWO use, along with improved lung compliance, arterial blood gases, and reduced pulmonary infections after physiotherapy.

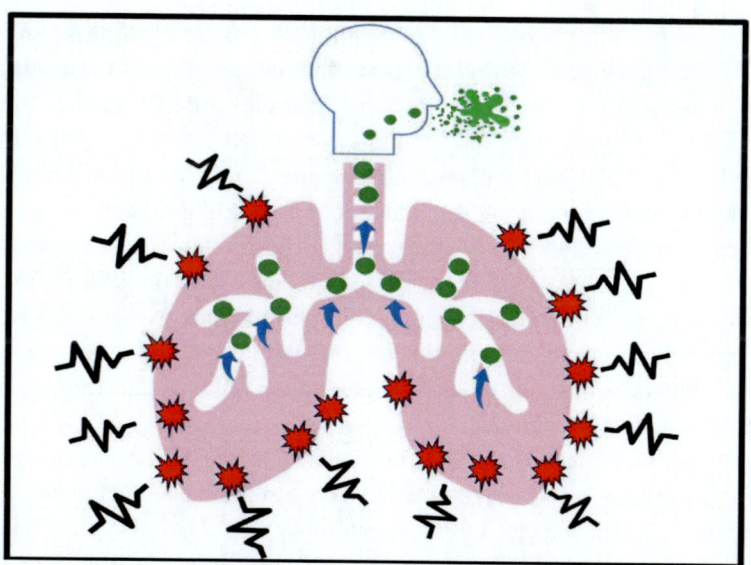

Figure 4. Effect of HFCWO. High-frequency oscillation (Black lines) exert a percussion effect (red icons) on the lung parenchyma, causing movement of the mucus (green circles) from the peripheral airways to the central, up to the trachea with centripetal movement (blue arrow) allowing mucus expectoration.

In a study conducted by Piquet et al. 12 patients with severe and stable COPD were subjected to high-frequency chest wall oscillation (HFCWO) at 5 Hz using an inflatable vest [26]. The researchers compared gas exchange and breathing patterns during both control periods and HFCWO periods, each lasting 15 minutes. The findings revealed that there was no change in Minute Ventilation (MV), but the breathing pattern was significantly altered during HFCWO. The breathing frequency decreased from 18 ± 6 breaths per minute during the control period to 14 ± 5 breaths per minute, while the tidal volume increased from 600 ± 200 ml during the control period to 860 ± 400 ml. As a result of these changes in the breathing pattern, the arterial oxygen pressure (PaO2) slightly increased from 54 ± 7 mm Hg during the control period to 57 ± 8 mm Hg during HFCWO, and the arterial carbon dioxide pressure (PaCO2) significantly decreased from 46 ± 6 mm Hg during the control period to 43 ± 7 mm Hg during HFCWO. Additionally, the duty cycle of breathing (Ti/Ttot, where Ti is inspiratory time and Ttot is the total duration of a breath) decreased from 0.37 ± 0.03 s during the control period to 0.29 ± 0.05 s during HFCWO. The researchers also observed a significant decrease in the TTdi index (Tension-time index, which assesses respiratory muscle function) from 0.06 ± 0.03 during the control period to 0.04 ± 0.02 during HFCWO. This decrease in the duty cycle suggests that inspiratory muscle work was facilitated under HFCWO. Based on these results, the research team suggests that HFCWO may be beneficial for patients with severe COPD in terms of both gas exchange and inspiratory muscle function. Perry et al. [27] demonstrated that adding positive end-expiratory pressure (PEEP) to high-frequency chest wall oscillation (HFCWO) at 10 Hz, with a mean chest wall pressure of 16 cm of water, increased end-expiratory lung volume and mean oscillatory flow rates during inspiration and expiration in patients with COPD. They suggested that PEEP should be used in conjunction with HFCWO to maximize sputum clearance with this technique.

Jones and Rowe et al. [28] stated that none of the bronchopulmonary hygiene methods have been reported to have a significant effect on respiratory functions in patients with COPD and bronchiectasis. They also mentioned that the studies included in their review were not sufficient to determine which patient subgroups might benefit. The authors suggested that there is not enough evidence to determine whether bronchopulmonary hygiene techniques are supportive or inadequate in patients with acute or stable COPD, chronic bronchitis, or bronchiectasis. In a randomized, multi-center, double-masked phase II clinical trial, Mahajan et al. [29] studied 52 participants who were randomized to either active (n = 25) or sham (n = 27) treatment. The study analyzed the use of HFCWO (High-Frequency Chest Wall Oscillation) early in the treatment of adults hospitalized for acute asthma or chronic obstructive pulmonary disease (COPD). Patients received active or sham treatment for 15 minutes three times a day for a total of four treatments, with medical management standardized across both groups.

The primary outcomes measured were patient adherence to therapy after four treatments (measured in minutes used out of 60 minutes prescribed) and patient satisfaction. The secondary outcomes included the change in Borg dyspnea score (with a change of ≥ 1 unit indicating a clinically significant change), spontaneously expectorated sputum volume, and forced expired volume in 1 second.

Both groups showed high levels of patient adherence and satisfaction. After four treatments, a higher proportion of patients in the active treatment group experienced a clinically significant improvement in dyspnea. However, there were no significant differences in the other secondary outcomes.

The researchers concluded that HFCWO is well tolerated in adults hospitalized for acute asthma or COPD and significantly improves dyspnea. They also mentioned that the high levels of patient satisfaction in both treatment groups justify the need for sham controls when evaluating the use of HFCWO on patient-reported outcomes. Chakravorty et al. conducted a randomized controlled crossover pilot study comparing HFCWO with conventional treatment. The study recruited 22 patients with moderate to severe COPD and mucus hypersecretion. Patients spent 4 weeks using HFCWO and 4 weeks in a conventional phase with a 2-week washout. Eleven patients started with HFCWO and changed to conventional treatment, while the other eleven started with conventional treatment and crossed over to HFCWO.

The patients were elderly and were at the upper end of the normal range of body mass index. The majority of patients had moderate to severe COPD, with a mean percentage predicted forced expiratory volume in 1 second of 41 (SD 15.6) and percentage predicted forced vital capacity of 73 (SD 17.7). Baseline sputum production was negatively correlated to lung function and positively correlated to St George's Respiratory Questionnaire. Symptom scores and St George's Respiratory Questionnaire symptom dimension improved significantly; sputum production showed a declining trend in the HFCWO phase, although the change did not reach statistical significance. The HFCWO device was well tolerated with good reported compliance. The authors concluded that the study demonstrated that patients with advanced COPD and mucus hypersecretion, who are at increased risk of declining lung function, tolerated the HFCWO treatment well. This led to an improvement in quality of life and reduced symptoms.

Nicolini et al. conducted a study to investigate whether adding IPV or HFCWO to the best pharmacological therapy (PT) would offer additional clinical benefit over chest physiotherapy in patients with severe COPD [31]. Sixty patients were randomly assigned to three groups: IPV group (treated with PT and IPV), PT group (treated with PT and HFCWO), and control group (treated with PT alone). The primary outcome measures included the dyspnea scale (modified Medical Research Council) and the Breathlessness, Cough, and Sputum scale (BCSS), as well as an evaluation of daily life activity (COPD Assessment Test [CAT]). Secondary outcome measures were pulmonary function testing, arterial blood gas analysis, and hematological examinations. Additionally, sputum cell counts were performed at the beginning and at the end of the study.

The results revealed that patients in both the IPV group and the HFCWO group exhibited significant improvement in dyspnea and daily life activity evaluations (modified Medical Research Council scale, BCSS, and CAT) compared to the control group, as well as in pulmonary function tests (forced vital capacity, forced expiratory volume in 1 second, forced expiratory volume in 1 second/forced vital capacity%, total lung capacity, residual volume, diffusing lung capacity monoxide, maximal inspiratory pressure, maximal expiratory pressure) and arterial blood gas values. However, when comparing the IPV group and the HFCWO group, a significant improvement in the IPV group was observed in maximal inspiratory pressure, maximal expiratory pressure, BCSS, and CAT. Similar results were seen in changes of sputum cytology with a reduction of inflammatory cells (neutrophils and macrophages).

The researchers concluded that both techniques improved daily life activities and lung function in patients with severe COPD. IPV demonstrated significantly greater effectiveness in improving some pulmonary function tests related to the small bronchial airways obstruction, respiratory muscle strength, and scores on health status assessment scales (BCSS and CAT) as well as a reduction of sputum inflammatory cells compared with HFCWO. Huang et al. conducted a review and meta-analysis of randomized controlled trials (RCTs) to assess the effectiveness of high-frequency chest wall oscillation (HFCWO) in helping patients with acute exacerbations of chronic obstructive pulmonary disease (COPD) expectorate sputum and reduce their hospital length of stay [32]. The study also looked into the impact of HFCWO on pulmonary function and oxygenation. The researchers used the PRISMA methodology and statistical analysis software to evaluate the risk of bias. Out of 5439 articles identified, 13 studies involving 756 patients were included in the meta-analysis. The results showed that compared to other airway clearance techniques, HFCWO led to a significant increase in expected sputum volume by 6.18 mL and a reduction in hospital stay by 4.37 days. However, there were no significant improvements in FEV1 (%), PaO2, and PaCO2. The researchers concluded that patients experiencing acute exacerbations of COPD may benefit from HFCWO therapy, as it helps them clear more sputum and shorten their hospital stays. In a recent study, Li Li et al. conducted a prospective, randomized controlled trial to investigate the effectiveness and safety of using piperacillin-tazobactam in combination with high-frequency chest-wall oscillation (HFCWO) for treating pneumonia in patients with acute exacerbation of chronic obstructive pulmonary disease (ECOPD). The researchers randomly assigned 92 patients with ECOPD and pneumonia to either an intervention group or a control group. The control group received standard treatment with oxygen, antibiotics, antispasmodics, antiasthmatic drugs, and mucolytic drugs, along with HFCWO for sputum removal. In addition to these treatments, the intervention group received piperacillin-tazobactam.

The study measured the treatment's efficacy one day after the intervention and assessed pulmonary function, laboratory indexes, and blood gas analysis at baseline and one day post-intervention. The researchers recorded the time until clinical symptoms disappeared, including cough, sputum, dyspnea, and pulmonary rales, calculated the length of hospital stay, and evaluated the treatment's safety.

The results showed that the intervention group had significantly higher clinical efficacy than the control group. The intervention group also had shorter durations of cough, sputum expulsion, dyspnea, disappearance of pulmonary rales, and hospitalization compared to the control group.

Furthermore, both groups showed improved pulmonary function post-intervention, with the intervention group demonstrating significantly higher improvement compared to the control group. Additionally, levels of certain markers such as IL-2, IL-10, TNF-α, CRP, and PCT decreased post-intervention, with the intervention group showing significantly lower levels than the control group.

In terms of safety, the intervention group had a lower incidence of adverse reactions compared to the control group, with only one participant reporting a decreased appetite. The study concluded that combining piperacillin-tazobactam with HFCWO for sputum evacuation can effectively treat patients with pneumonia and exacerbation of COPD with high safety, making it a treatment worthy of clinical application.

COPD and bronchiectasis are prevalent conditions in the general population. The frequency of bronchiectasis among COPD patients has been examined in numerous studies, yielding varying results from 4% to 72% [34, 35, 36]. Bronchiectasis in COPD has been linked to lower body mass index, older age, increased sputum production and purulence, more comorbidities, airflow obstruction, dyspnea, and reduced exercise capacity [37, 38, 39].

In a study involving 30 patients diagnosed with bronchiectasis using high resolution computed tomography, ten patients received bronchial cleansing therapy twice daily for 15 days over a 5-day week. Traditional chest physiotherapy was administered to 10 patients for 45 minutes per day, while high-frequency chest wall oscillation (HFCWO) at 13-15 Hz frequency was provided to another 10 patients. The remaining 10 patients received only medical treatment. Results indicated a decrease in the inflammatory marker C-reactive protein level and improvements in forced vital capacity and forced expiratory volume in 1 second (FEV1) for the patient group receiving HFCWO [40].

Most studies on the high-frequency chest wall oscillation technique have involved a limited number of patients. One study, which evaluated approximately 2596 patients, analyzed hospitalization rates, antibiotic use, and quality of life criteria from the records of bronchiectasis patients undergoing HFCWO treatment before and after. The findings demonstrated a decrease in hospitalization rates due to respiratory issues from 49.1% to 24.0% after HFCWO treatment. Moreover, the ability to clear the lungs, a primary goal of HFCWO treatment, increased from 13.9% to 76.6%. The study concluded that this physiotherapy technique significantly improved secretion excretion [41].

Contraindications

Absolute contraindications for HFCWO include unstable head and neck trauma, active hemorrhage, hemoptysis, and respiratory distress syndrome. Relative contraindications are suspected cases of tuberculosis, chest pain, acute bronchospasm, subcutaneous emphysema, recent epidural or spinal infusion, skin burns, infection, graft, recently placed transvenous catheter or subcutaneous pacemaker, recent thoracic or abdominal surgery, rib fracture, and osteomyelitis [24].

These patients require close monitoring in cases of respiratory failure, as they may experience decreased oxygen saturation during acute exacerbation or in the presence of pneumonia.

The procedure should not be applied to intensive care patients with newly inserted gastrostomy tubes. It is also important to prevent vomiting during or after the procedure in mechanically ventilated patients. Therefore, it is recommended to perform the procedure 1 hour before or 2 hours after nasogastric tube feeding [25].

Conclusion

The modern HFCWO physiotherapy technique has been shown in several studies to offer significant advantages in terms of its efficiency and application compared to conventional physiotherapy. Patients with conditions such as cystic fibrosis, bronchiectasis, ciliary dyskinesia syndrome, lung cavity diseases, pulmonary muscle dysfunction, and neuromuscular diseases, as well as those who cannot use other airway clearance techniques, have been treated with this technique.

The mechanism of action of HFCWO physiotherapy results in increased mucus excretion by creating expiratory flow higher than inspiratory flow, similar to a normal cough. This helps in clearing the peripheral bronchial tree, facilitating mucus expectoration, increasing mucus volume, and improving oxygenation while reducing respiratory fatigue and infections.

The positive effects on the body include improvements in respiratory mechanics and exchanges. This includes a decrease in respiratory frequency, an increase in tidal volume, an increase in end-expiratory lung volume, improved lung compliance, and overall improvement in arterial blood gas analysis with increased arterial Po_2 and decreased arterial pCO_2. Furthermore, the work of the inspiratory muscles is significantly facilitated. Additionally, pulmonary function tests show improvement and a reduction in sputum inflammatory cells and CRP has been observed.

In patients with exacerbation of COPD, the combination of the antibiotics piperacillin/tazobactam with HFCWO therapy has been found effective in improving mucociliary clearance and reducing hospital stays with high safety. The respiratory therapy parameters can be adjusted using relevant monitors depending on the type of device used.

Therapy cycles involve a combination of the following factors: oscillation frequency ranging from 2 to 25 HZ, which corresponds to the speed of compressions; vest pressure ranging from 1 to 10; duration of pauses; and the percentage of compression of the device, which can range from 10% to 100%. The therapy should be administered twice a day for 20-30 minutes, and in more severe cases, every 3-4 hours a day per cycle. The use of PEEP is recommended and should be used in conjunction with HFCWO to enhance sputum removal and reduce mucus production, thus lowering the risk of lung infections. This approach has shown particular benefits in advanced COPD and individuals with mucus hypersecretion, as well as those at increased risk of lung function decline such as ECOPD. Patients have demonstrated high adherence and satisfaction, and the therapy is well tolerated by hospitalized adults as well as those receiving home care, due to its easy autonomous management and simple application. In conclusion, the application of HFCWO results in improved lung function, reduced symptoms, faster recovery, and a return to daily activities, ultimately enhancing quality of life.

Key Messages

1. HFCWO is a modern physiotherapy technique characterized by a wearable vest and a device to set the parameters.
2. HFCWO involves high-frequency oscillations on the chest wall, which helps in releasing mucus by increasing expectoration.
3. HFCWO has been shown to improve inflammatory indices in sputum.
4. HFCWO has been found to be as effective as traditional physiotherapy.
5. HFCWO can also be used for uncooperative patients.
6. HFCWO can be managed independently by the patient and therefore can be used at home.

References

[1] Anzueto, A., Cohen, M., Echazarreta, A. L., et al. Delphi Consensus on Clinical Applications of GOLD 2023 Recommendations in COPD Management: How Aligned are Recommendations with Clinical Practice?. *Pulmonary Therapy* 2024 Mar;10(1):69-84.

[2] Petty, T. L., et al. The history of COPD. *International Journal of Chronic Obstructive Pulmonary Disease* 2006;1(1):3-14.

[3] Pahal, P., Avula, A., Sharma, S. *Emphysema*. In: StatPearls [Internet]. Treasure Island (FL): StatPearls Publishing; 2024 Jan-. Available from: https://www.ncbi.nlm.nih.gov/books/NBK482217.

[4] Lozano, R., Naghavi, M., Foreman, K., et al. Global and regional mortality from 235 causes of death for 20 age groups in 1990 and 2010: a systematic analysis for the Global Burden of Disease Study *2010*. *The Lancet* 2012, Dec 15;380(9859):2095-128.

[5] Gregory A. Roth et al. GBD 2017 Causes of Death Collaborators. Global, regional, and national age-sex-specific mortality for 282 causes of death in 195 countries and territories, 1980-2017: a systematic analysis for the Global Burden of Disease Study. *Lancet* 2018;392:1736–1788.

[6] Soriano, J. B., Abajobir, A. A., Abate, K. H., et al. Global, regional, and national deaths, prevalence, disability-adjusted life years, and years lived with disability for chronic obstructive pulmonary disease and asthma, 1990–2015: a systematic analysis for the Global Burden of Disease Study. *The Lancet Respiratory Medicine* 2017 Sep;5(9):691-706.

[7] Mirza, S., Clay, R. D., Koslow, M. A., & Scanlon, P. D. COPD Guidelines: A Review of the 2018 GOLD Report. *Mayo Clinic Proceedings* 2018 Oct;93(10):1488-1502.

[8] Vestbo, J., Papi, A., Corradi, M., et al. Single inhaler extrafine triple therapy versus long-acting muscarinic antagonist therapy for chronic obstructive pulmonary disease *(TRINITY):* a double-blind, parallel group, randomised controlled trial. *The Lancet* 2017 May 13;389(10082):1919-1929.

[9] Wedzicha, J. A., Calverley, P. M. A., Albert, R. K., et al. Management of COPD exacerbations: a European Respiratory Society/American Thoracic Society guideline. *The European Respiratory Journal* 2017 Mar 15;49(3):1600791.

[10] Ram, F. S. F., Picot, J., Lightowler, J., et al. Non-invasive positive pressure ventilation for treatment of respiratory failure due to exacerbations of chronic obstructive pulmonary disease. *Cochrane Database of Systematic Reviews* 2004:(3):CD004104.

[11] Ninane, V., Geltner, C., Bezzi, M., et al. Multicentre European study for the treatment of advanced emphysema with bronchial valves. *The European Respiratory Journal* 2012 Jun;39(6):1319-25.

[12] Sciurba, F. C., Criner, G. J., Strange, C., et al. Effect of Endobronchial Coils vs Usual Care on Exercise Tolerance in Patients With Severe Emphysema. *JAMA* 2016 May;315(20):2178-89.

[13] Celli, B. R., Fabbri, L. M., Aaron, S. D., et al. An Updated Definition and Severity Classification of Chronic Obstructive Pulmonary Disease Exacerbations: The Rome Proposal. *American Journal of Respiratory and Critical Care Medicine* 2021 Dec 1;204(11):1251-1258.

[14] Donaldson, G. C., et al. Relationship between exacerbation frequency and lung function decline in chronic obstructive pulmonary disease. *Thorax* 2002 Oct;57(10):847-52.

[15] Miravitlles, M., et al. Effect of exacerbations on quality of life in patients with chronic obstructive pulmonary disease: a 2 year follow up study. *Thorax* 2004 May;59(5):387-95.

[16] Vollenweider, D., Jarrett, H., Steurer-Stey, C. A., et al. Antibiotics for exacerbations of chronic obstructive pulmonary disease. *The Cochrane Library* 2012 Dec 12:12:CD010257.

[17] Brochard, L., Mancebo, J., Wysocki, M., et al. Noninvasive Ventilation for Acute Exacerbations of Chronic Obstructive Pulmonary Disease. *The New England Journal of Medicine* 1995 Sep 28;333(13):817-22.

[18] Bhowmik, A., Chahal, K., Austin, G., et al. Improving mucociliary clearance in chronic obstructive pulmonary disease. *Respiratory Medicine* 2009 Apr;103(4):496-502.

[19] Leemans, G., Belmans, D., Van Holsbeke, C., et al. The effectiveness of a mobile high-frequency chest wall oscillation (HFCWO) device for airway clearance. *Pediatr Pulmonol* 2020 Aug;55(8):1984-1992.

[20] Oermann, C. M., Swank, P. R., & Sockrider, M. Validation of an Instrument Measuring Patient Satisfaction With Chest Physiotherapy Techniques in Cystic Fibrosis. *Chest* 2000 Jul;118(1):92-7.

[21] Darbee, Joan C., Kanga, Jamshed F., Ohtake, Patricia J., Physiologic evidence for high-frequency chest wall oscillation and positive expiratory pressure breathing in hospitalized subjects with cystic fibrosis. *Physical Therapy* 2005 Dec;85(12):1278-89.

[22] King, M., Phillips, D. M., Gross, D, et al. Enhanced Tracheal Mucus Clearance with High-frequency Chest Wall Compression. *The American Review of Respiratory Disease* 1983 Sep;128(3):511-5.

[23] Scherer, TA., Barandun, J., Martinez, E., et al. Effect of high- frequency oral airway and chest wall oscillation and conventional chest physical therapy on expectoration in patients with stable cystic fibrosis. *Chest* 1998 Apr;113(4):1019-27.

[24] Kermenli, Tayfun. Respiratory care and non invasive ventilation. Airway secretions devices. In Book Respiratory care in Non-invasive Mechanical Ventilator support. Principles and Practice, edited by Antonio M. Esquinas, Mohammed D. Alahmari. Nova Science Publishers, Inc. 2021:177-182.

[25] Esguerra-Gonzales, A., Ilagan-Honorio, M., Kehoe, P., et al. Effect of high-frequency chest wall oscillation versus chest physiotherapy on lung function after lung transplant. *Applied Nursing Research* 2014 Feb;27(1):59-66.

[26] Piquet, J., Brochard, L., Isabey, D., et al. High-frequency Chest Wall Oscillation in Patients wih Chronic Air-Flow Obstruction. *The American Review of Respiratory Disease* 2022 Jun;54(2):150-156.

[27] Perry, R. J., Man, G. C., & Jones, R. L. Effects of Positive End-Expiratory Pressure on Oscillated Flow Rate During High-Frequency Chest Compression. *Chest* 1998 Apr;113(4):1028-33.

[28] Jones, A., & Rowe, B. H. Bronchopulmonary hygiene physical therapy for chronic obstructive pulmonary disease and bronchiectasis. *Cochrane Database of Systematic Reviews* 2000:(2):CD000045.

[29] Mahajan, A., Diette, G. B., Hatipoğlu, U., et al. High-frequency chest wall oscillation for asthma and chronic obstructive pulmonary disease exacerbations: a randomized sham-controlled clinical trial. *Respiratory Research* 2011 Sep 10;12(1):120.

[30] Chakravorty, I., Chahal, K., & Austin, G. A pilot study of the impact of high-frequency chest wall oscillation in chronic obstructive pulmonary disease patients with mucus hypersecretion. *International Journal of Chronic Obstructive Pulmonary Disease* 2011:6:693-9.

[31] Nicolini, A., Grecchi, B., Ferrari-Bravo, M., et al. Safety and effectiveness of the high-frequency chest wall oscillation vs intrapulmonary percussive ventilation in patients with severe COPD. *International Journal of Chronic Obstructive Pulmonary Disease* 2018 Feb 16:13:617-625.

[32] Huang, H., Chen, K. H., Tsai, C. L., et al. Effects of High-Frequency Chest Wall Oscillation on Acute Exacerbation of Chronic Obstructive Pulmonary Disease: A Systematic Review and Meta-Analysis of Randomized Controlled Trials. *International Journal of Chronic Obstructive Pulmonary Disease* 2022 Nov 10:17:2857-2869.

[33] Li, Li, Feng, Q., et al. Efficacy and Safety Analysis of Piperacillin Tazobactam in Combination With High-frequency Chest Wall Oscillation in Patients With COPD Coupled With Pneumonia. *Altern Ther Health Med* 2023 Jan;29(1):124-129.

[34] Bafadhel, M. The Role of CT Scanning in Multidimensional Phenotyping of COPD. *Chest* 2011 Sep;140(3):634-642.

[35] Gallego, M., Pomares, X., Espasa, M., et al. Pseudomonas aeruginosa isolates in severe chronic obstructive pulmonary disease: characterization and risk factors. *BMC Pulmonary Medicine* 2014 Jun 26:14:103.

[36] Gonçalves, J. R., Corso Pereira, M., Figueiras Pedreira De Cerqueira, E. M., et al. Severe obstructive disease: Similarities and differences between smoker and non-smoker patients with COPD and/or bronchiectasis. *Revista Portuguesa De Pneumologia* 2013 Jan-Feb;19(1):13-8.

[37] Patel, I., Vlahos, I., Wilkinson, T. M. A., et al. Bronchiectasis, Exacerbation Indices, and Inflammation in Chronic Obstructive Pulmonary Disease. *American Journal of Respiratory and Critical Care Medicine* 2004 Aug 15;170(4):400-7.

[38] Jeffrey I. Stewart, Maselli, D. J., Anzueto, A., et al. Clinical impact of CT radiological feature of bronchiectasis in the COPDGene cohort. *American Journal of Respiratory and Critical Care Medicine* 2012;185:A3656.

[39] Gatheral, T., Kumar, N., Sansom, B., et al. COPD-related Bronchiectasis; Independent Impact on Disease Course and Outcomes. *COPD: Journal of Chronic Obstructive Pulmonary Disease* 2014 Dec;11(6):605-14.

[40] Nicolini, A., Cardini, F., Landucci, N., et al. Effectiveness of treatment with high-frequency chest wall oscillation in patients with bronchiectasis. *BMC Pulmonary Medicine* 2013 Apr 4:13:21.

[41] Barto, T. L., Maselli, D. J., Daignault, S., et al. Real-life experience with high-frequency chest wall oscillation vest therapy in adults with non-cystic fibrosis bronchiectasis. *Therapeutic Advances in Respiratory Disease* 2020 Jan-Dec:14:1753466620932508.

Chapter 13

High-Frequency Chest Wall Oscillation in Neuromuscular Pulmonary Disorders

Elvia Giovanna Battaglia[1,*], MD
Elena Compalati[2], MD
Salvatore Sciurello[2], MD
Giuseppe Russo[2], MD
and Paolo Innocente Banfi[2], MD

[1]Respiratory Unit, Neuromuscular OmniCentre (NeMO),
Neurorehabilitation, University of Milan, Niguarda Hospital, Milan, Italy
[2]UOC Riabilitazione Cardiorespiratoria,
Fondazione Don Carlo Gnocchi-IRCCS Santa Maria Nascente, Milan, Italy

Abstract

Patients with complex neuromuscular disorders (cNMD) are at risk of reduced vital capacity due to weakness in inspiratory muscles and changes in the lungs and chest wall mechanical properties. As a result, cNMD patients including those with neuromuscular disease and cerebral palsy, have airway clearance difficulties, due also to mobilization deficit, which may cause aspiration, respiratory infection, and death. Upper-airway obstruction syndromes, reflux and aspiration of gastric contents, impaired lower-respiratory secretion clearance due to weak cough, frequent lower-respiratory-tract infections, chest wall deformities and related deformities of the tracheobronchial tree contribute to morbidity and represent a constant challenge to clinicians. The presence of NMD, motor neuron disease and respiratory muscle weakness increase the

---

[*] Corresponding Author's Email: ebattaglia@dongnocchi.it.

In: High-frequency Chest Wall Oscillation Therapy in Critical Ill Patients
Editor: Antonio M. Esquinas
ISBN: 979-8-89530-264-4
© 2025 Nova Science Publishers, Inc.

probability of pulmonary complications, morbidity, and mortality in this population; furthermore, secretion retention is common in these patients and is primarily due to the inability to generate an effective cough, with secondary stasis of bronchial secretions and reduction of airway clearance and muco-ciliary function. For this reason, to promote clearance of these lower respiratory secretions, chest physical therapy is often incorporated into the management of patients with neurological impairment. The selection of chest physical therapy methods, used in this group of patients, depends on several factors, like the cognitive status of the patient and the severity of respiratory impairment. In this chapter, we wanted to carry-out a state-of-the-art review, regarding high-frequency chest wall oscillation (HFCWO) and its use in adult patients affected by neuromuscular diseases.

Keywords: high-frequency chest wall oscillation (HFCWO), intrapulmonary percussive ventilation, airway clearance techniques, mucociliary clearance impairment, neuromuscular disorders

Introduction

Most neuromuscular diseases (NMDs) are characterized by progressive muscular impairment leading to ambulation loss, becoming wheelchair-bound, swallowing difficulties, respiratory muscle weakness, and, eventually, death from respiratory failure [1]. Rapidly progressive NMDs, such as amyotrophic lateral sclerosis (ALS) and spinal muscular atrophies (SMA), are characterized by muscle impairment, which worsens over months and results in death within a few years. A relatively rapid progression is seen in Duchenne muscular dystrophy (DMD), leading in muscle impairment and a significantly reduced life expectancy, with death possibly occurring in young adulthood. Other myopathies, such as Becker muscular dystrophy, facioscapulohumeral muscular dystrophy, limb-girdle muscular dystrophy and myotonic dystrophy, experience a slowly progressive reduction in muscular function and only a mildly reduced life expectancy [2].

A reduction in inspiratory muscle strength associated with ineffective alveolar ventilation, expiratory muscle weakness and impaired airway secretion clearance can lead to life threatening problems and respiratory failure, which is the most common cause of morbidity and mortality for patients affected by chronic or rapidly progressive NMDs. The muscular components of the respiratory system are:

1. The inspiratory muscles (diaphragm, scalene and external intercostal) that contribute most to ventilation.
2. The expiratory muscles carry-out forced expiration and expulsive efforts including coughing.
3. The bulbar muscles that protect the airways [2].

Due to progressive inspiratory muscle weakness and increasing elastic load induced by reduced lung and thorax compliance, resulting in an increased work of breathing (WOB), these patients suffer from a progressive decline in vital capacity (VC). A rapid–shallow breathing pattern may be associated with increased work of breathing and an inability to take deep breaths, leading to chronic micro atelectasis and decreased lung and chest wall compliance [3]. NMDs may also be associated with obstructive or central sleep-disordered breathing, particularly during rapid eye movement sleep (REM). In this condition, respiratory muscle weakness and/or mechanical disadvantage depending on the involvement of upper airway muscles and respiratory center neurons (e.g., in myotonic dystrophy) [4] and comorbidities, such as obesity may result in severe alveolar hypoventilation leading to sustained oxygen desaturation and hypercapnia [5]. Due to the patient's difficulty in moving, dyspnea usually has a late onset through the disease evolution. Thus, lung function and respiratory muscle function monitoring should be mandatory, as both are considered to be the best prognostic indicators in these patients [6]. Respiratory muscle impairment leads to impaired coughing and difficulty on clearing respiratory secretions, with subsequent mucous plugging and a raised risk of pulmonary infections. These events are a prominent source of healthcare needs, comprising prolonged hospitalizations and the use of costly medical devices [7].

Patients with complex neuromuscular disorders (cNMD) are at risk of reduced vital capacity due to weakness in inspiratory muscles and changes in the lungs and chest wall mechanical properties [8]. As a result, cNMD patients including those with neuromuscular disease and cerebral palsy, have airway clearance difficulties, also due to mobilization deficit, which may lead to aspiration, respiratory infection, and death. Upper-airway obstruction syndromes, reflux and aspiration of gastric contents, impaired lower-respiratory secretion clearance due to weak cough, frequent lower-respiratory-tract infections, chest wall deformities and related deformities of the tracheobronchial tree contribute to morbidity and represent a constant challenge to clinicians [9]. Respiratory complications are the leading cause of morbidity and mortality in patients with NMDs and respiratory muscle weakness; secretion retention is common in these patients and is primarily due to an inability to generate an effective cough [10].

Compromised cough is common in many primary neurologic conditions and spinal cord injuries, but patients with spinal cord injuries (SCI) may also suffer from mucus hypersecretion and an increase in bronchial tone. In cervical spinal cord injuries, parasympathetic overstimulation resulting from sympathetic denervation to the lungs leads to an abnormal quantity and quality of mucus in the initial stages following injury. Effective cough requires full pre-cough inspiration, followed by glottis closure and adequate expiratory muscle strength to generate sufficient intra-thoracic pressures, to obtain high peak expiratory flows. This cough expiratory airflow can be measured and is known as peak cough flow (PCF). Expiratory muscle weakness combined with inadequate lung inflation prevents effective coughing and airway clearance altering airway resistance and increasing the risk of developing atelectasis and pneumonia. Bulbar muscle weakness (facial, oropharyngeal and laryngeal muscles) can affect the ability to speak, swallow and clear airway secretions, with the possibility of an increased likelihood of aspiration. Drooling is an indicator of severe swallowing impairment. Patients with NMDs usually experience mild-to-moderate bulbar dysfunction except for patients with ALS, type 1 SMA and other rapidly progressive NMD, who may develop a severe glottis functional impairment. The presence of NMD, motor neuron disease and respiratory muscle weakness increase the probability of pulmonary complications, morbidity and mortality in this population; furthermore, secretion retention is common in these patients and is primarily due to the inability to generate an effective cough, with secondary stasis of bronchial secretions and reduction of airway clearance and muco-ciliary function.

For this reason, chest physical therapy is often incorporated into the management of patients with neurological impairment to promote the clearance of lower respiratory secretions.

Intrapulmonary percussive ventilation (IPV) therapy has shown to be effective in adolescents and adults with neuromuscular diseases [11]. Other chest physical therapy modalities include end-expiratory positive pressure devices, manual chest physical therapy, high-frequency chest wall compression (HFCWC) and high-frequency chest wall oscillation (HFCWO). The selection of chest physical therapy methods for this group of patients, depends on several factors, such as the cognitive status of the patient and the severity of respiratory impairment [12]. Noah Lechtzin et al. conducted a study with the aim to determine if HFCWO therapy leads to improved outcomes as measured by lower healthcare use for patients, who have a chronic neuromuscular disease [7]. They demonstrated that total allowed medical costs and inpatient hospitalization costs were less in the period after initiation of HFCWO than before initiation. Fitzgerald et al. demonstrated that long-term HFCWC may reduce the number of hospitalizations and hospitalization days in children with neurological impairment and pulmonary infections [12]. HFCWC should be considered as an important part of the complex approach to respiratory health in children with neurological impairment and chronic respiratory disorders. At least Ansaripour et al. lead a budget impact analysis that showed HFCWO is a cost-saving strategy in managing cNMD [13]. The reduction in hospitalization costs offset additional costs of the HFCWO device (Vest TM System). Future research efforts should be devoted to further defining the indications for HFCWC in separate groups of patients with neurological impairment, depending on their diagnosis, cognitive function, and degree of respiratory impairment.

In this chapter, we wanted to carry out a state-of-the-art review, regarding high-frequency chest wall oscillation (HFCWO) and its use in adult patients affected by neuromuscular diseases.

Pathophysiology Mucociliary Clearance Impairment

Airway clearance depends on ciliary beat coordination and power, cough peak flow, and the rheological properties of secretions. Effective mucus clearance is essential for lung health and a consistent consequence of poor clearance often leads to airway diseases, such as neuromuscular diseases. Healthy mucus is a gel with low viscosity and elasticity that is easily transported by ciliary action, whereas pathologic mucus has higher viscosity and elasticity and is less easily cleared [14]. The conversion from healthy to pathologic mucus occurs by multiple mechanisms that change its hydration and biochemical constituents. These include abnormal secretion of salt and water, increased production of mucins, infiltration of mucus with inflammatory cells, and heightened broncho-vascular permeability. The accumulation of mucus results from some combination of overproduction, decreased clearance and persistent accumulation, which can lead to infection and inflammation by providing an environment for microbial growth [15]. Various aerosolized medications have been used to improve airway clearance by altering mucus biophysical properties in healthy individuals, but there is no clinical pieces of evidence on the use of these medications in patients affected by neuromuscular diseases, as demonstrated by a systematic review made by the American Association for Respiratory Care in 2015 [10]. this review found that evidence from randomized controlled trials (RCTs) was weak and insufficient to support the use of medications to improve airway clearance, oxygenation, ventilator time, hospital stay, change sputum properties, improve quality of life, or respiratory mechanics compared with usual care [10-16]. Although some organizations have recommended nonpharmacologic airway clearance therapies, only two guidelines recommend the use of inhaled medication for this purpose [18-19]. However, the American College of Chest Physicians' practice guidelines on pharmacologic pro-tussive therapy, specifically state that these medications should not be prescribed to promote airway clearance in patients with NMD or impairment [20]. In healthy individuals, mucociliary clearance and cough mechanisms are effective and efficient in defending against secretion encumbrance, but these mechanisms may become ineffective in case of system malfunction and/or excessive bronchial secretions. Mucus is normally transported under normal circumstances from the lower respiratory tract into the pharynx by cephalad-bias airflow and the mucociliary escalator mechanism [21].

Weakness of inspiratory muscles leads to a progressive decrease in vital capacity (VC), but the lung volume changes observed in some patients with neuromuscular disorders (NMDs) are attributable to a combination of muscle weakness and alterations in the mechanical properties of the lungs and chest wall [22]Severe bulbar dysfunction and glottic dysfunction most commonly occur in patients with amyotrophic lateral sclerosis (ALS), spinal muscle atrophy (SMA) type 1, other rare neuromuscular disorders, such as x-linked myotubular myopathy and pseudobulbar palsy of central nervous system etiology [23]. Glottis and vocal cords incompetence results in complete loss of the ability to cough and swallow. Difficulty swallowing liquids may result in pooling of saliva and mucus in the pharynx, especially in the valleculate and the pyriform sinuses. This results in the perception of excessive pharyngeal secretions, similar to post-nasal drip [24]. Although mucus clearance is preserved in NMD [25], patients with chronic respiratory infections from aspiration or retained secretions may develop a cycle of infection and inflammation that can impair ciliary function, cause airway remodeling, and alter the physical properties of secretions [15]. Infants and children have chest-wall instability, lower functional residual capacity, and smaller airway diameter, providing additional challenges for clearing airway secretions, even in the absence of diseases that impair cough reflexes [26]. Nowadays patients with NMDs have a longer life expectancy [8] and consequently, we are seeing more complex ventilator-dependent patients.

Respiratory physiotherapy is an essential part of the multi-disciplinary management of these individuals [8]. However, due to the the inherent heterogeneity of the condition and the growing number of available airway clearance techniques (ACTs) and associated technological developments, it is challenging for doctors and physical therapists to determine which assessments and treatment options are more appropriate for people with NMD. ACTs for people affected by NMDs can be classified into proximal (cough augmentation) and peripheral (secretion mobilizing). Details are provided in Table 1.

Table 1. Classification of airway clearance techniques used in patients affected by neuromuscular diseases [8]

Airway Clearance Techniques available for Respiratory Physiotherapy
PROXIMAL ACT's "COUGH AUGMENTATION"
1. Assisted Inspiration
• *Single breaths*
– Mechanical insufflation
– Non-Invasive Ventilation (NIV)
– Intermittent positive Pressure Breathing (IPPB)
• *Stacked breaths*
– Air Stacking (AS)
– Glossopharyngeal Breathing (GPB)
– Volume Cycled NIV
– Lung Volume Recruitment Bag
– Resuscitation Bag with Patient Holding their Breath
2. Assisted Expiration
• Manual Assisted Cough (MAC)
• Mechanical Exsufflation
3. Assisted Inspiration and Expiration
• Any combination of Assisted Inspiration and Assisted Expiration Techniques
• Mechanical Insufflation-Exsufflation (MI-E)
• PERIPHERAL ACT's "SPUTUM MOBILIZING"
• Manual Techniques (MT)
• High-Frequency Chest Wall Oscillation (HFCWO)
• High-Frequency Chest Wall Compression (HFCWC)
• Intrapulmonary Percussive Ventilation (IPV)
• Chest Wall Strapping (CWS)

Mucus impacted in the small and basilar airways can lead to atelectasis and ease the development of chest infection [27]. High-frequency chest wall oscillation (HFCWO) devices apply pressure to the chest wall accompanied by high-frequency vibration, which been shown to move secretions from peripheral airways toward more central airways. This is an accepted approach to secretion clearance in neuromuscular disease (15), but the evidence supporting HFCWO comes largely from case studies, case series, and a few small clinical trials [28-29].

In the scientific literature, there are also interesting *in vitro* studies about tracheal mucus clearance in high-frequency oscillation therapy. These studies highlighted that:

1. High-frequency ventilation by rapid chest wall compression enhances tracheal mucus clearance compared to spontaneous breathing, whereas high-frequency oscillation at the mouth does not [30]
2. There is a positive correlation between viscoelasticity and spinnability and a negative correlation between spinnability and the cough clearability index (CCI), but no correlation between spinnability and the mucociliary clearability index (MCI). Oscillating airflow seemed to act as a physical "mucolytic," that affected mostly the cough clearability of the mucus simulant [31].

HFCWO/C Indications in Neuromuscular Disorders

There is limited data on the efficacy of high-frequency chest wall compression (HFCWC) therapy in adults with neurological impairment and very few data on the impact of HFCWC on healthcare costs in this category of patients. Other chest physical therapy modalities include end-expiratory positive pressure devices, manual chest physical therapy and high-frequency chest wall oscillation (HFCWO). The selection of one method or another for use in this group of patients depends on several factors, previously enhanced in this chapter [12]. Yuan and co-workers [32] investigated HFCWC in patients with NMD; their data suggest that HFCWC is safe, well-tolerated, and has better compliance compared to "standard chest physiotherapy." Crescimanno and Marrone suggested that HFCWC is easy to use and accepted by patients with NMDs [28]. They showed improvements in clinical and radiological condition and suggested that it was helpful for patients with scoliosis, in whom conventional respiratory physiotherapy is not possible. HFCWC has been shown to decrease the work of breathing and the sensation of breathlessness in patients with ALS and a sub-group showed a decreased rate of FVC decline [7].

A case report of HFCWO in severely unwell NIV-dependent patient with type 1 spinal muscular atrophy suggested that the device was safe, and the

Authors concluded that the increase in ventilator-free time was attributed to improved secretion clearance [33]. However, there is also the potential to mobilize a large quantity of secretions into the central airways, with the potential to precipitate respiratory arrest. The major limitations of this technique in patients with NMD is that proximal ACT's and ventilator support could be needed to clear secretions from the central airways. Therefore, it is essential to have equipment readily available to clear secretions from the airway [8]. The devices are also expensive, compared to other methods of ACT's. HFCWO/C should be considered an important part of the complex approach to respiratory health in children with neurological impairment and chronic respiratory disorders. These devices in people with NMD should be used in combination with ventilator support. Future research efforts should be devoted to further defining the indications for HFCWO/C in different groups of patients with neurological impairment, depending on their diagnosis, cognitive function, and degree of respiratory impairment.

Clinical Practice Recommendations in Neuromuscular Pulmonary Disorders

From the data published in the literature we propose these recommendations:

1. Positive expiratory pressure (PEP) and oscillatory PEP devices: people with neuromuscular disorders (NMD) generally cannot generate sufficient expiratory flow for the technique to be effective. Therefore, we do not recommend these devices for patients with NMD. Peripheral Airway Clearance Techniques (ACTs) aim to improve ventilation, loosen secretions, and enhance mucus transport from peripheral airways to the central airways (12th generation of the bronchial tree and above), with higher expiratory than inspiratory airflows (called biased expiratory flow).
2. HFCWO, or compression (HFCWC), intrapulmonary percussive ventilation (IPV): the physiologic effects on mucus clearance relates to generation of air-liquid shear forces. The eccentric flow pattern (higher expiratory flow than inspiratory flow) may promote transport of secretions centrally and reduces mucus viscosity [8].

$$OCI = f \times \frac{T_I}{T_E} \times \frac{\dot{V}_{E\text{-}max}}{\dot{V}_{I\text{-}max}} - f$$

Abbreviations: OCI = oscillatory clearance index, f = oscillatory frequency (Hz), TI = duration of outward inspiratory airway wall displacement, TE = duration of inward expiratory airway wall displacement, V̇ E-max = maximum expiratory flow, and V̇ I-max = maximum inspiratory flow.

Figure 1. Classification of airway clearance techniques used in patients affected by neuromuscular diseases (modified from Chatwin et al 2018) [8].

Based on theoretical considerations from previous studies, Scherer et al. [34] developed a mathematical model to identify optimal settings for mucus transport Figure 1.

The higher the Oscillatory Clearance Index (OCI), the faster the rate of mucus transport. This model confirms that the greater the expiratory flow compared to the inspiratory flow, the quicker the movement towards the inside of the wall of the airways during exhalation.

King et al. found a frequency-dependent reduction in viscosity with oscillations from 3 Hz to 16 Hz [30]. However, other researchers found an increase in viscosity with oscillations from 1 Hz to 8 Hz. Tomkiewicz et al. observed that viscosity decreased after 30 min of oscillation at a frequency of 22 Hz [31]. Vibration of the chest wall might stimulate the vagus nerve through reflex pathways in the airway walls or in the chest wall. Mechanical resonance (possibly in the range of 11–15 Hz) may increase the strength of the ciliary beat. This suggests that in people with NMDs it's good practice to use the highest frequency tolerated by the patient (without causing fatigue), that produces an increase in PEF relative to PIF.

The use of these techniques is possible in infants, children, and adults, even in the presence of a tracheostomy, bulbar failure or intellectual impairment [8]. As with all peripheral ACT's, in individuals with neuromuscular disorders it is essential to ensure effective proximal ACT's, to prevent secretion retention in the central airways.

These techniques should be used in conjunction with ventilator support when the Vital Capacity (VC) is low or when the subject reports fatigue during performance. In the literature there are no clear indications on when to use NIV orhow to modify its settings. It may be necessary to increase ventilatory support or other parameters during the use of the corset or armor precisely because these represent an increased load on the chest. Alternatively, the literature [8-35] shows that Intrapulmonary Percussive Ventilation (IPV) therapy is effective in adolescents and adults with neuromuscular disease dependent on ventilators. However, lower frequencies and higher pressures can support patient ventilation (Figure 2).

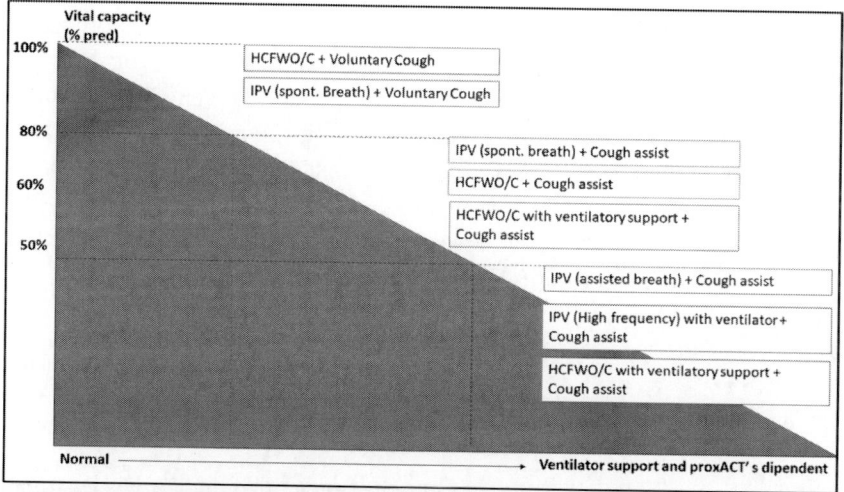

Figure 2. Proximal and distal ACT'S strategies based on Vital Capacity reduction and ventilatory support increase in order to maintain a proper Airway clearance Technique. Particularly, through a worsening of the clinical conditions (reduction of VC and a proportional rise on Ventilatory Support) there are different ACTs that can be taken into account to ensure a correct airway clearance.

The starting frequency for this device is equal to 5 Hz, building up to 10–15 Hz. There have been no studies evaluating treatment times or frequencies in NMD. Therefore, treatments are individualized or based on manufactures pre-set programs. Often treatments in NMD are around 5-30 min stages or until the patient feels the need to cough using proximal ACT's or experiences significant fatigue. HCFWO treatment can be performed two to several times a day.

Conclusion

Most neuromuscular diseases (NMDs) are characterized by progressive inspiratory muscle strength associated with ineffective alveolar ventilation, expiratory muscle weakness and impaired airway secretion clearance This can lead to life-threatening problems and respiratory failure. Secretion retention is common in these patients and is primarily due to the inability to generate an effective cough, resulting in secondary stasis of bronchial secretions and reduction of airway clearance and muco-ciliary function.

For this reason, chest physical therapy is often incorporated into the management of patients with neurological impairment to promote the clearance of lower respiratory secretions. The selection of the most appropriate chest physical therapy method depends on several factors, such as the cognitive status of the patient and the severity of respiratory impairment. HFCWO/C should be considered as an important part of the complex approach to respiratory health in people with NMD and should be used in combination with ventilator support. Future research efforts should be devoted to further defining the indications for HFCWO in different groups of patients with neurological impairment.

Key Messages

1. In neuromuscular disorders a reduction in inspiratory muscle strength associated with ineffective alveolar ventilation, expiratory muscle weakness and impaired airway secretion clearance can lead to respiratory failure.
2. Respiratory muscle impairment leads to impaired coughing and difficulty on clearing respiratory secretions, with subsequent mucous plugging and a raised risk of pulmonary infections.
3. Intrapulmonary percussive ventilation (IPV) therapy has shown to be effective in adolescents and adults with neuromuscular diseases.
4. HFCWO should be considered as an important part of the complex approach to respiratory health in patients with neurological impairment and chronic respiratory disorders.

References

[1] Hill M, Hughes T, Milford C. Treatment for swallowing difficulties (dysphagia) in chronic muscle disease. *Cochrane Database Syst Rev* 2004;(2):CD004303.
[2] Ambrosino N, Carpenè N, Gherardi M. Chronic respiratory care for neuromuscular diseases in adults. *Eur Respir J* 2009;34(2):444-451.
[3] Goldstein NA Roger S, ed. *Ventilatory Support for Chronic Respiratory Failure*. CRC Press; 2013.

[4] Culebras A. Sleep and neuromuscular disorders. *Neurol Clin* 2005;23(4):1209-1223.

[5] Ono S, Takahashi K, Kanda F, et al. Decrease of neurons in the medullary arcuate nucleus in myotonic dystrophy. *Acta Neuropathol* 2001;102(1):89-93.

[6] Toussaint M, Steens M, Soudon P. Lung function accurately predicts hypercapnia in patients with Duchenne muscular dystrophy. *Chest* 2007;131(2):368-375.

[7] Lechtzin N, Wolfe LF, Frick KD. The Impact of High-Frequency Chest Wall Oscillation on Healthcare Use in Patients with Neuromuscular Diseases. *Ann Am Thorac Soc* 2016;13(6):904-909.

[8] Chatwin M, Toussaint M, Gonçalves MR, et al. Airway clearance techniques in neuromuscular disorders: A state of the art review. *Respir Med* 2018;136:98-110.

[9] Birnkrant DJ. New challenges in the management of prolonged survivors of pediatric neuromuscular diseases: A pulmonologist's perspective. *Pediatric Pulmonology* 2006;41(12):1113-1117.

[10] Strickland SL, Rubin BK, Haas CF, Volsko TA, Drescher GS, O'Malley CA. AARC Clinical Practice Guideline: Effectiveness of Pharmacologic Airway Clearance Therapies in Hospitalized Patients. *Respiratory Care* 2015;60(7):1071-1077.

[11] Chatwin M, Ross E, Hart N, Nickol AH, Polkey MI, Simonds AK. Cough augmentation with mechanical insufflation/exsufflation in patients with neuromuscular weakness. *Eur Respir J* 2003;21(3):502-508.

[12] Fitzgerald K, Dugre J, Pagala S, Homel P, Marcus M, Kazachkov M. High-frequency chest wall compression therapy in neurologically impaired children. *Respir Care* 2014;59(1):107-112.

[13] Ansaripour A, Roehrich K, Mashayekhi A, et al. Budget Impact of the Vest™ High-frequency Chest Wall Oscillation System for Managing Airway Clearance in Patients with Complex Neurological Disorders: A US Healthcare Payers' Perspective Analysis. *Pharmacoecon Open* 2022;6(2):169-178.

[14] Cone RA. Barrier properties of mucus. *Adv Drug Deliv Rev* 2009;61(2):75-85.

[15] Fahy JV, Dickey BF. Airway mucus function and dysfunction. *N Engl J Med* 2010;363(23):2233-2247.

[16] Sathe NA, Krishnaswami S, Andrews J, Ficzere C, McPheeters ML. Pharmacologic Agents That Promote Airway Clearance in Hospitalized Subjects: A Systematic Review. *Respir Care* 2015;60(7):1061-1070.

[17] Miller RG, Jackson CE, Kasarskis EJ, et al. Practice parameter update: the care of the patient with amyotrophic lateral sclerosis: drug, nutritional, and respiratory therapies (an evidence-based review): report of the Quality Standards Subcommittee of the American Academy of Neurology. *Neurology* 2009;73(15):1218-1226.

[18] Birnkrant DJ, Bushby KMD, Amin RS, et al. The respiratory management of patients with duchenne muscular dystrophy: a DMD care considerations working group specialty article. *Pediatr Pulmonol* 2010;45(8):739-748.

[19] Bott J, Blumenthal S, Buxton M, et al. Guidelines for the physiotherapy management of the adult, medical, spontaneously breathing patient. *Thorax* 2009;64 Suppl 1:i1-51.

[20] Bolser DC. Cough suppressant and pharmacologic protussive therapy: ACCP evidence-based clinical practice guidelines. *Chest* 2006;129(1 Suppl):238S-249S.

[21] Fink JB. Forced expiratory technique, directed cough, and autogenic drainage. *Respir Care* 2007;52(9):1210-1221; discussion 1221-1223.
[22] Bach JR. Noninvasive ventilation is more than mask ventilation. *Chest* 2003;123(6):2156-2157; author reply 2157.
[23] Chaudri MB, Liu C, Hubbard R, Jefferson D, Kinnear WJ. Relationship between supramaximal flow during cough and mortality in motor neurone disease. *Eur Respir J* 2002;19(3):434-438.
[24] Elman LB, Dubin RM, Kelley M, McCluskey L. Management of oropharyngeal and tracheobronchial secretions in patients with neurologic disease. *J Palliat Med* 2005;8(6):1150-1159.
[25] Finder JD. A 2009 perspective on the 2004 American Thoracic Society statement, "respiratory care of the patient with Duchenne muscular dystrophy." *Pediatrics* 2009;123 Suppl 4:S239-241
[26] Oberwaldner B. Physiotherapy for airway clearance in paediatrics. *Eur Respir J* 2000;15(1):196-204.
[27] Kallet RH. Adjunct therapies during mechanical ventilation: airway clearance techniques, therapeutic aerosols, and gases. *Respir Care* 2013;58(6):1053-1073.
[28] Crescimanno G, Marrone O. High-frequency chest wall oscillation plus mechanical in-exsufflation in Duchenne muscular dystrophy with respiratory complications related to pandemic Influenza A/H1N1. *Rev Port Pneumol* 2010;16(6):912-916.
[29] Lange DJ, Lechtzin N, Davey C, et al. High-frequency chest wall oscillation in ALS: an exploratory randomized, controlled trial. *Neurology* 2006;67(6):991-997.
[30] M King, D M Phillips, A Zidulka, et al. Tracheal mucus clearance in high-frequency oscillation. II: Chest wall versus mouth oscillation. Am Rev Respir Dis. 1984 Nov;130(5):703-6.
[31] Tomkiewicz RP, Biviji A, King M. Effects of oscillating air flow on the rheological properties and clearability of mucous gel simulants. *Biorheology* 1994;31(5):511-520.
[32] Yuan N, Kane P, Shelton K, Matel J, Becker BC, Moss RB. Safety, tolerability, and efficacy of high-frequency chest wall oscillation in pediatric patients with cerebral palsy and neuromuscular diseases: an exploratory randomized controlled trial. *J Child Neurol* 2010;25(7):815-821.
[33] Keating JM, Collins N, Bush A et al. High-Frequency Chest-Wall Oscillation in a Noninvasive-Ventilation-Dependent Patient With Type 1 Spinal Muscular Atrophy. Respir Care 2011 Nov;56 (11):1840-3
[34] Scherer TA, Barandun J, Martinez E, Wanner A, Rubin. EM. Effect of high-frequency oral airway and chest wall oscillation and conventional chest physical therapy on expectoration in patients with stable cystic fibrosis. *Chest* 1998;113(4).
[35] Toussaint M, Chatwin M, Gonzales J, Berlowitz DJ, ENMC Respiratory Therapy Consortium. 228th ENMC International Workshop: Airway clearance techniques in neuromuscular disorders Naarden, The Netherlands, 3-5 March, 2017. *Neuromuscul Disord* 2018;28(3):289-298.

Chapter 14

High-Frequency Chest Wall Oscillation for Ventilator-Associated Pneumonia

Hılal Sıpahıoglu*, MD
Department of Intensive Care, Kayseri Education and Research Hospital, Kayseri, Turkey

Abstract

Ventilator-associated pneumonia (VAP) is a type of hospital-acquired pneumonia that occurs in patients who have been on mechanical ventilation with an endotracheal tube or tracheostomy for more than 48 hours. The most critical risk factor for the development of pneumonia is invasive mechanical ventilation. Both hospital-acquired pneumonia (HAP) and ventilator-associated pneumonia pose significant public health challenges due to their high mortality and morbidity rates. For intensive care specialists, preventing HAP, particularly VAP, is of paramount importance. Effective prevention strategies focus on addressing key aspects of the disease's pathogenesis, such as facilitating the movement of secretions from the periphery to the center in intubated patients. High-frequency chest wall oscillation (HFCWO) aids in this process by promoting the movement of secretions toward the center, allowing for easier aspiration and reducing peak pressures. Research indicates that HFCWO not only lowers the risk of pneumonia but also shortens the length of stay in intensive care and reduces the duration of mechanical ventilation. Since prolonged mechanical ventilation and extended intensive care stays increase the risk of VAP, preventing its development is vital. Additionally, minimizing the need for invasive mechanical ventilation in patients with bronchiectasis and cystic fibrosis can indirectly reduce the risk of VAP.

---

* Corresponding Author's Email: hilalgul1983@gmail.com.

In: High-frequency Chest Wall Oscillation Therapy in Critical Ill Patients
Editor: Antonio M. Esquinas
ISBN: 979-8-89530-264-4
© 2025 Nova Science Publishers, Inc.

Keywords: ventilator-associated pneumonia, prevention, high-frequency chest wall oscillation, invasive mechanical ventilation, sputum expectoration

Definition and Incidence

Hospital-acquired pneumonia (HAP) is an infection affecting lung parenchyma, caused by pathogens that are present in the hospital environment [1]. When pneumonia develops 48 hours or after a patient is admitted to the hospital, it is classified as hospital-acquired pneumonia. HAP is the second most common nosocomial infection and is the leading cause of death among critically ill patients due to hospital-acquired infections. Ventilator-associated pneumonia (VAP) is a specific type of hospital-acquired pneumonia that occurs in patients with endotracheal tubes or tracheostomies who have been on mechanical ventilation for over 48 hours. Both hospital-acquired pneumonia and ventilator-associated pneumonia are major public health issues due to their high mortality and morbidity rates. A meta-analysis has shown that VAP is responsible for 32.5% of average mortality in ICU patients. Ventilator-associated pneumonia significantly extends the duration of ICU and hospital stays, as well as the time that the patient requires respiratory support [1, 2]. The most critical risk factor for HAP is intubation. Mechanical ventilation is an essential life-saving intervention for critically ill patients, with approximately 300,000 individuals in the United States connected to mechanical ventilation on a daily bases [3]. This condition also accounts for more than half of the antibiotics prescribed in the ICU and contributes to the rising cost of hospitalization, with the average cost attributed to the disease ranging between 2089.13€ and >29431.70€. Consequently, the search for preventive measures to reduce these parameters and prevent the onset of the disease has become crucial [2, 4, 5].

Pathogenesis

The normal human respiratory tract is protected by a variety of defense mechanisms against infection. These include anatomical barriers such as the glottis and larynx, reflexes like coughing, components in tracheobronchial secretions, mucociliary clearance, epithelial lining fluid, surfactant components, cell-mediated and humoral immunity, and a phagocytic system involving alveolar macrophages and recruited neutrophils. Both humoral and cell-mediated adaptive immunity also play essential roles. When these components work together effectively, invading pathogens are eliminated, preventing the development of clinical disease. However, if these defenses are compromised, or overwhelmed by a high load of organisms or those with unusual virulence, pneumonitis can occur. As evidenced by the rare association of ventilator associated pneumonia with bacteremia, many of these diseases are thought to result from the aspiration of potential pathogens that colonize the mucosal surfaces of the oropharyngeal airways, dental plaque, and/or paranasal sinuses. Endotracheal intubation disrupts the natural barrier between the oropharynx and trachea, allowing contaminated secretions to enter the lungs directly through the subglottic space and past the endotracheal tube valves. In intubated patients, contaminated secretions can exacerbate by lying in a supine position. Additionally, biofilm formation on the inner and outer surfaces of the endotracheal tube creates a protected environment for pathogens. Aggregates from the biofilm that are released during aspiration pose a significant threat to the lungs, as they are difficult to clear by the host's immune defenses and are destroyed by antibiotics [6-8].

Diagnosis

Ventilator-associated pneumonia (VAP) is linked to increased morbidity, extended hospital stays, higher healthcare costs, and elevated mortality rates, making its prevention a crucial objective. The diagnosis of VAP can be summarized by three key elements: a) Clinical signs indicative of infection, such as the new onset of fever, purulent sputum, leukocytosis, increased minute ventilation, a decline in arterial oxygenation, and/or the need for increased vasopressor infusion to maintain blood pressure, b) new or progressive persistent radiographic opacities c) "positive" microbiologic culture results for a potentially pathogenic microorganism isolated from tracheal aspirates, bronchoalveolar lavage (BAL) fluid, pleural fluid, and/or blood.

The primary causes of ventilator-induced lung injury in mechanically ventilated patients include impaired clearance of airway secretions, edema due to changes in pulmonary capillary permeability, respiratory muscle weakness acquired in the intensive care unit, and alterations in lung compliance.

Table 1. Risk factors of VAP [1]

Risk factors of VAP related with the host	Risk factors of VAP related with hospitalization process	Risk factors of VAP related with drug therapy
- Advanced age - Burns - Chronic or preexisting pulmonary disease (tuberculosis, chronic obstructive pulmonary disease, [b]bronchiolitis) - Cigarette smoking - Coma - Gastric colonization - Immunosuppressive disease[a] - Impaired consciousness - Male gender - Malnutrition - Neurological/neuromuscular disease - Organ failure - Oropharynx colonization - Post-operative acute respiratory failure - Post-surgical - Post-traumatic - Septicemia - Sinusitis - Trauma[c] - Underlying disease, and its severity	- Bronchoscopy - Emergency intubation[b] - Endotracheal intubation - Enteral nutrition - Frequent changes of the ventilator circuit - Gastric aspiration[b] - High-frequency of antibiotic resistance in the hospital unit where the patient is hospitalized[a] - Hospitalization ≥ 5 days[a] - Long-term hospital and ICU length of stay. - Long-term intubation - Mechanical ventilation - Multiple central venous lines [b] - Nasogastric tube - Re-intubation[c] - Supine body position - Thoracic surgery - Tracheostomy[c] - Transportation from ICU to other hospital sites	- Antacids[c] - Antibiotic therapy in the previous 90 days[a] - Excessive sedation - H2-receptor antagonists - Imunosupressive drugs (corticosteroids)[a] - Intravenous sedatives[b] - Neuromuscular blockers - Prior exposure to antibiotics, particularly to third-generation cephalosporins - Proton pump inhibitors - Red blood cells transfusions (immunomodulatory effects) - Stress ulcer prophylaxis

a: Risk factor for multidrug-resistant pathogens.
b: Specific risk factors of early-onset VAP.
c: Specific risk factors of late-onset VAP.

It is estimated that 8% to 28% of patients on mechanical ventilation develop pneumonia, with the risk being 3 to 10 times higher compared to non-ventilated patients. Moreover, around 90% of nosocomial pneumonia cases in the intensive care unit occur during mechanical ventilation. The development of pneumonia is influenced by a variety of risk factors, which are categorized into three groups, as outlined in Table 1.

Prevention

Preventing Hospital-Acquired Pneumonia, particularly Ventilator-Associated Pneumonia, is a top priority for intensive care specialists. Effective prevention requires targeted interventions in the critical aspects of the disease's pathogenesis, which can be systematically addressed. General infection control is essential in preventing HAP/VAP, including strict adherence to universal hand hygiene, meticulous decontamination of respiratory therapy equipment, and appropriate patient isolation. Prevention of VAP begins with evaluating the necessity for invasive mechanical ventilation. The most effective strategy for preventing VAP is to minimize the duration of mechanical ventilation. The risk of VAP increases with each additional day on mechanical ventilation, rising sharply after seven days. Consequently, strategies that encourage the early discontinuation of mechanical ventilation are crucial. Research has demonstrated that daily sedation interruptions and daily spontaneous breathing trials can significantly reduce the duration of ventilation.

Avoiding mechanical ventilation whenever possible is essential. Daily spontaneous breathing trials, the most widely used method for weaning from mechanical ventilation, should be performed to monitor for signs of respiratory failure. Since reintubation is a significant risk factor for VAP, making accurate extubating decisions and ensuring proper post-extubation care are critical.

Cough function plays a critical role in clearing secretions, but effective coughing may be compromised in patients undergoing endotracheal intubation, mechanical ventilation, and sedation. As a result, these patients may accumulate large amounts of pulmonary secretions, which can worsen bronchial hygiene, oxygen-hemoglobin saturation, ventilation-perfusion matching, and lead to lung atelectasis or collapse. Intratracheal intubation and mechanical ventilation can impair muco-ciliary clearance, cause secretion retention, and deteriorate lung conditions, increasing the risk of reintubation if spontaneous breathing trials are unsuccessful.[9]

VAP prevention strategies are shown in Table 2.

Conventional chest physical therapy (CCPT) can aid in dislodging airway secretions. However, in severe cases, more advanced airway clearance techniques (ACT) are needed to effectively clear secretions and support the rehabilitation of respiratory function. ACT, such as high-frequency chest wall oscillation (HFCWO), is widely used in intensive care units worldwide to assist in clearing airway secretions.

Research has demonstrated that multiple daily sessions of HFCWO can more effectively increase the concentration of surfactant protein in the alveoli. This enhancement of surfactant protein suggests that HFCWO can reduce pulmonary capillary permeability, lower alveolar surface tension, improve static lung compliance, and help mitigate various lung injuries caused by mechanical ventilation, including ventilator-induced lung injury.

Table 2. VAP prevention strategies

Basic practices	Special approaches	Generally not recommended
Avoid intubation if possible (NIMV)	Selective oral or digestive decontamination	Silver-coated endotracheal tubes
Minimize sedation 1. Manage ventilated patients without sedatives whenever possible 2. Interrupt sedation once a day (spontaneous awakening trials) for patients without contraindications 3. Assess readiness to extubate once a day (spontaneous breathing trials) in patients without contraindications 4. Pair spontaneous breathing trials with spontaneous awakening trials	Regular oral care with chlorhexidine	Kinetic beds
Maintain and improve physical conditioning. (Provide early exercise and mobilization)	Prophylactic probiotics	Prone positioning
Minimize pooling of secretions above the endotracheal tube cuff	Ultrathin polyurethane endotracheal tube cuffs	Stress ulcer prophylaxis
Elevate the head of the bed	Automated control of endotracheal tube cuff pressure	Early tracheotomy
Maintain ventilator circuits	Saline instillation before tracheal suctioning	Monitoring residual gastric volumes
	Mechanical tooth brushing	Early parenteral nutrition

High-frequency chest wall oscillation (HFCWO) mimics a "mini-cough" by compressing and relaxing the chest wall to generate oscillatory airflow through the lungs, effectively displacing airway secretions in a manner comparable to conventional chest physical therapy (CCPT), while reducing the manpower required for CCPT. In a study by Chuang et al. involving intubated pneumonia patients, Ppeak values significantly decreased in those who underwent HFCWO [10].

Additionally, the study referenced demonstrated that the use of High-Frequency Chest Wall Oscillation (HFCWO), compared with Chest Physiotherapy (CPT), led to significant improvements in various parameters among elderly patients without non-cystic fibrosis as summarized in Table 3 [11].

Table 3. Parameters associated with improvement in chest phsyotherapy

1. Blood Inflammation Parameters: (Significant improvements in C-reactive protein levels were observed).
2. Lung Functionality: (Positive effects on lung functionality were noted, indicating potential benefits for respiratory health)
3. Dyspnea: (Reduction in dyspnea (shortness of breath) was observed, suggesting an improvement in respiratory symptoms).
4. Quality of Life Scales: (Positive changes were noted in quality of life scales, indicating an overall enhancement in the well-being of the elderly patients).

High-frequency chest wall oscillation (HFCWO) is an effective early rehabilitation strategy for enhancing lung function in patients on mechanical ventilation. In a study by Liu and colleagues, the use of HFCWO during acute exacerbations of Chronic Obstructive Pulmonary Disease (COPD) was shown to reduce the duration of mechanical ventilation, a critical factor in lowering the risk of Ventilator-Associated Pneumonia (VAP) [12].

Conclusion

Although no studies have directly demonstrated that HFCWO reduces the incidence of VAP, it may help prevent pneumonia in intubated patients by mobilizing secretions from the periphery to the central airways, making them easier to aspirate and reduce peak airway pressures. Research also shows that HFCWO can shorten both the duration of intensive care stays and mechanical ventilation. Since the risk of developing VAP increases with prolonged mechanical ventilation and extended ICU stays, HFCWO could indirectly reduce this risk. Furthermore, by decreasing the need for invasive mechanical ventilation in patients with bronchiectasis and cystic fibrosis, HFCWO may further lower the risk of VAP.

Key Messages

1. Hospital-acquired pneumonia (HAP) and ventilator-associated pneumonia (VAP) are major public health concerns due to their high mortality and morbidity rates.

2. Effective prevention of HAP and VAP requires targeting critical aspects of their pathogenesis and should be systematically implemented.
3. The first step in preventing VAP is to evaluate the necessity of invasive mechanical ventilation.
4. The risk of developing VAP increases with the duration of mechanical ventilation and extended stays in intensive care.
5. HFCWO may aid in preventing VAP by mobilizing secretions from the periphery to the center, making aspiration easier, improving mechanical ventilation, and reducing ICU stay duration.

References

[1] Oliveira J, Zagalo C, Cavaco-Silva P: Prevention of ventilator-associated pneumonia. *Rev Port Pneumol* 2014, 20(3):152-161.
[2] Rello J, Ollendorf DA, Oster G, Vera-Llonch M, Bellm L, Redman R, Kollef MH, Group VAPOSA: Epidemiology and outcomes of ventilator-associated pneumonia in a large US database. *Chest* 2002, 122(6):2115-2121.
[3] Magill SS, Klompas M, Balk R, Burns SM, Deutschman CS, Diekema D, Fridkin S, Greene L, Guh A, Gutterman D et al. Developing a new, national approach to surveillance for ventilator-associated events: executive summary. *Clin Infect Dis* 2013, 57(12):1742-1746.
[4] Erbay RH, Yalcin AN, Zencir M, Serin S, Atalay H: Costs and risk factors for ventilator-associated pneumonia in a Turkish university hospital's intensive care unit: a case-control study. *BMC Pulm Med* 2004, 4:3.
[5] Muscedere JG, Martin CM, Heyland DK: The impact of ventilator-associated pneumonia on the Canadian health care system. *J Crit Care* 2008, 23(1):5-10.
[6] Safdar N, Crnich CJ, Maki DG: The pathogenesis of ventilator-associated pneumonia: its relevance to developing effective strategies for prevention. *Respir Care* 2005, 50(6):725-739; discussion 739-741.
[7] Diaconu O, Siriopol I, Polosanu LI, Grigoras I: Endotracheal Tube Biofilm and its Impact on the Pathogenesis of Ventilator-Associated Pneumonia. *J Crit Care Med (Targu Mures)* 2018, 4(2):50-55.
[8] Chastre J, Fagon JY: Ventilator-associated pneumonia. *Am J Respir Crit Care Med* 2002, 165(7):867-903.
[9] Konrad F, Schreiber T, Brecht-Kraus D, Georgieff M: Mucociliary transport in ICU patients. *Chest* 1994, 105(1):237-241.
[10] Chuang ML, Chou YL, Lee CY, Huang SF: Instantaneous responses to high-frequency chest wall oscillation in patients with acute pneumonic respiratory failure receiving mechanical ventilation: A randomized controlled study. *Medicine (Baltimore)* 2017; 96(9):e5912.

[11] Nicolini A, Cardini F, Landucci N, Lanata S, Ferrari-Bravo M, Barlascini C: Effectiveness of treatment with high-frequency chest wall oscillation in patients with bronchiectasis. *BMC Pulm Med* 2013, 13:21.

[12] Liu T, Kang Y, Xu Z, Lyu Y, Jia L, Gao Y: [A study of the value of high-frequency chest wall oscillation in patients with acute exacerbation of chronic obstructive pulmonary disease]. *Zhonghua Jie He He Hu Xi Za Zhi* 2014, 37(4):255-259.

Chapter 15

High-Frequency Chest Wall Oscillation for Cystic Fibrosis Exacerbations in Pediatrics

Mariana Celiz Alonso[*], PT
Unit of Physical Therapy at Ricardo Gutierrez Children Hospital,
Pediatric and Neonatal Kinesiology Postgraduate Courses, Buenos Aires City, Argentina

Abstract

Cystic fibrosis (CF) is a chronic, progressive disease that mainly affects the respiratory and digestive systems.

Cystic fibrosis (CF) constitutes a significant burden in pediatric health and exacerbations represent critical events which impair respiratory function and quality of life. The management of exacerbations in cystic fibrosis is of vital importance to improve the quality of life of patients and prevent serious complications. Exacerbations in cystic fibrosis have a significant impact on patients' quality of life. These exacerbations can lead to impaired lung function, increased respiratory symptoms, frequent hospitalizations and decreased ability to perform daily activities.

There exist various techniques for airway mucociliary clearance including mechanical devices, physical therapies, breathing control exercises such as conventional chest physiotherapy techniques (CCPT), cyclic breathing techniques (ACBT), such as chest expansion, positive expiratory pressure therapy (PEP), oscillating airway devices (AOD), and airway management techniques (AOD). Standard HFCWO is a commonly prescribed ACT and consists of an inflatable vest that applies small volume expiratory pulses to the external chest wall, generating high-velocity expiratory airflow that is thought to mobilize secretions by the sheer force created. In conclusion, HFCWO emerges as a promising

---

[*] Corresponding Author's Email: marianaceliz@gmail.com.

In: High-frequency Chest Wall Oscillation Therapy in Critical Ill Patients
Editor: Antonio M. Esquinas
ISBN: 979-8-89530-264-4
© 2025 Nova Science Publishers, Inc.

technique for managing CF exacerbations in pediatrics, offering advantages in secretion clearance and respiratory function. However, challenges and controversies, including device availability and cost, emphasize the need for ongoing research to optimize its application and explore complementary techniques for comprehensive care. This chapter addresses the specific application of High-Frequency Chest Wall Oscillation (HFCWO) technology in the management of CF exacerbations in children, exploring its therapeutic potential.

Keywords: cystic fibrosis, high-frequency chest wall oscillation, pediatric, physiotherapy techniques, airway clearance techniques

Introduction

Cystic fibrosis (CF) is a chronic, progressive disease that mainly affects the respiratory and digestive systems [1]. It is an inherited disease caused by mutations in the CFTR gene, which regulates ion transport in epithelial cells. This genetic alteration leads to the production of abnormal, thick secretions in the lungs, pancreas and other organs, resulting in airway obstruction, recurrent infections and pancreatic dysfunction. The management of exacerbations in cystic fibrosis is of vital importance to improve the quality of life of patients and prevent serious complications. Cystic fibrosis (CF) constitutes a significant burden in pediatric health, and exacerbations represent critical events that affect respiratory function and quality of life. This chapter addresses the specific application of High-Frequency Chest Wall Oscillation (HFCWO) technology in the management of CF exacerbations in children, exploring its therapeutic potential. There are several techniques for the mucociliary clearance, including mechanical devices, physical therapies, breathing control exercises such as conventional chest physiotherapy techniques (CCPT), cyclic breathing techniques (ACBT), such as chest expansion, positive expiratory pressure therapy (PEP), oscillating airway devices (AOD), and airway management techniques (AOD) and also percussive devices (MP) and external compression devices (HFCC, HFCWC, and HFCWO) [1, 2].

Standard HFCWO is a commonly prescribed ACT and consists of an inflatable vest that applies small volume expiratory pulses to the external chest wall, generating high-velocity expiratory airflow that is thought to mobilize secretions by the sheer force created.

Extra thoracic oscillations are generated by forces external to the respiratory system, e.g., high-frequency chest wall oscillation (HFCWO) [1]. HFCWO implies the use of an inflatable vest connected to a high-frequency machine, which frequency and intensity are set by operator to ensure the individual's comfort and ease. This type of device can also be called the Vest® or Hayek Oscillator.

Keywords for the search on main databases (PUBMED, SCIELO, LILACS, COCHRANE) were: "Chest Wall Oscillation" [Mesh] OR "Chest Wall Oscillations" OR "External Chest Wall Oscillation" OR "High-Frequency Chest Wall Oscillation" OR "High-frequency Chest Wall Oscillation" OR "High-Frequency Chest Compression" OR "High-frequency Chest Compression" OR "High-Frequency Chest Compressions" OR "High-Frequency Chest Wall Compression" OR "High-frequency Chest Wall" OR "High-frequency Chest Wall."

The content of this chapter was developed taking into account scientific evidence and clinical experience.

Cystic Fibrosis

Cystic fibrosis is an autosomal recessive disease caused by mutations/variations in the CFTR gene. CFTR protein (called anion channel) helps to maintain the water-electrolyte balance in epithelial membranes of diverse organs including the upper and lower airways, intestines, pancreas, biliary tree, cervix, vas deferens, sweat glands, etc.

CFTR is involved in the regulation of transepithelial ion transport and water–electrolyte homeostasis in many organ systems. As to sweat glands, CFTR normal activity renders the chloride ion absorption from primarily isotonic perspiration whereas in CF patients, CFTR dysfunction produces impaired chloride absorption by sweat-gland ducts with consequent high chloride concentration in sweat.

The consequences of this fluid imbalance in the lungs are thickened secretions and reduced mucociliary transport, resulting in mucus retention and plugging of airways. Mucus plugging alone can cause an inflammatory response in the airways even in the absence of pathogens. Mucus retention also favors recurrent and persistent bacterial infections with consecutively increased mucus production and inflammation, a cycle leading to the development of structural lung damage (bronchiectasis).

Impact of Exacerbations on Quality of Life

Exacerbations in cystic fibrosis have a significant impact on patients' quality of life. These exacerbations can lead to impaired lung function, increased respiratory symptoms, frequent hospitalizations and decreased ability to perform daily activities.

Fundamentals

The High-Frequency Chest Wall Oscillation belongs to the category of oscillatory devices. These devices bear an oscillatory component which may involve intra or extra thoracic (HFCWO) oscillations [2].

HFCWC provides compression of the chest wall at frequencies that are similar to the resonant frequency of the lung, between 5 and 20 Hz via an air pulse generator that delivers intermittent positive airflow into the vest. The starting frequency for this device is 5 Hz building up to 10-15 Hz [2]. Inflation and deflation of the vest produce a transient/oscillatory increase in the airflow of airways while vibrating secretions from peripheral airways towards mouth. Ventilator support may be jointly used.

HFCWO also provides compression of the chest wall at frequencies that are similar to the resonant frequency of the lungs via a negative pressure ventilator attached to a vest. As the ventilator delivers negative pressure the air is sucked into the lungs. When the negative pressure ceases the patient breathes out. The device has the ability to deliver high-frequency intermittent negative pressure on top of the patients spontaneous or NIV supported breathing. This also produces a transient/oscillatory increase in airflow in the airways vibrating the secretions from the peripheral airways toward the mouth.

The treatments are individualized or based on manufacturer's pre-set programs [3].

It has been shown that this sheer force changes rheology and moves mucus in a cephalic direction during the oscillation [4-5].

Mechanisms

The HFCWO provides several ways to improve secretion clearance in cystic fibrosis patients. Firstly, the high-frequency vibrations help to break down the viscosity of secretions, which facilitates their mobilization and expectoration. In addition, HFCWO promotes airway opening and lung expansion, which improves ventilation and oxygenation.

Various mechanisms of action have been proposed for HFCWO:

1. Augmentation of the expiratory flow, which increases the annular flow of mucus towards the oropharynx when exceeding by more than 10% the inspiratory peak flow [6].
2. Improvement of mucus rheological (spin ability and viscoelastic) properties.
3. Reflected stimulation of Vagus nerve promotes increase of ciliary motility, especially when applied oscillations range between 11 and 15hz, and
4. Enhancement of the gas-liquid transport

Advantages

Medical literature has studied the benefits of HFCWO in cystic fibrosis exacerbations in children. Some of the potential benefits include improved mobilization and clearance of lung secretions: The HFCWO technique uses high-frequency vibrations on the chest wall to help mobilize and expel lung secretions. This can facilitate airway clearance and improve lung function.

Reduction in exacerbation severity: The addition of HFCWO to medical treatment has been shown to decrease airway obstruction and benefit individuals with cystic fibrosis during acute respiratory exacerbations in the treatment of acute pulmonary exacerbation in adult cystic fibrosis (CF) patients [7]. Enhanced respiratory function: HFCWO promotes better airflow and ventilation, leading to improved oxygenation and overall respiratory health. Publications on HFCWO date back to 1987 where Piquet evaluated its impact on adult patients with obstructive pulmonary disease.

Only in 2002 Plioplys et al. in their case series evaluated its effect on children with cerebral palsy in an uncontrolled study. The authors observed that the variable effectiveness of suctioning improved before and after vest therapy (VT), a statistically significant difference. In 2009, one of the first reviews of the cystic fibrosis population was published by the Medical Advisory Secretariat of the Canadian Ministry of Health. Main and Rain [8] and Wilson [9] in their systematic reviews explored the existing evidence on the effectiveness of conventional chest physiotherapy versus other therapies including extrapulmonary mechanical percussion. There were no differences in rate of decline in FEV1 or FVC % predicted between the two techniques but the annual rate of decline in FEF25- 75 was greater in those using HFCC than those using CCP. Two short- term studies reported fewer days in hospital due to respiratory exacerbations in the extrapulmonary MP group, but there was no difference in time to first IV antibiotics between the groups in the long-term study.

There was no difference in adherence rate between the study groups [10], but the long-term study reported significantly lower treatment satisfaction scores in the CCP group compared to the HFCC group. Additional lung function tests were performed in only one short-term study and there were no differences after 14 days.

Assessment of quality of life (QoL) during the study was performed in only one long-term study and there were no differences between groups in the 12 health-related quality of life (HRQoL) domains. There were no differences in adherence rates between the groups in either the short- or long-term studies, but the long-term study reported significantly lower treatment satisfaction scores in the CCP group compared to the HFCC group.

In terms of other outcomes, studies reported heterogeneity in weight gain in the HFCC group compared to the CCP group. One short-term study measured mucus weight and found that sputum production was similar between groups after 24 hours. In addition, adverse events were reported in the short-term studies, such as hemoptysis, which resolved after 24 hours in one participant in the HFCC group and two participants in the CCPT group, as well as chest pain and nausea in some participants in the HFCC group.

Patient and Caregiver Training in the Proper Use Of HFCWO

Although currently there is a wider range of respiratory physiotherapy options, patients have found it difficult to sustain treatment over time. This is quite sound if we consider that these techniques consume a large amount of time per day limiting the patient to being at home and away from their normal social life. Studies have reported low adherence in all age groups (i.e., children [11-12], adolescents, and adults [13], with adherence declining as patients age and their daily routines become more complex [14].

Challenges and Controversies in the Use of HFCWO

Limitations and Possible Contraindications

Devices may not be readily available in some countries and are also expensive. Other important limitations are the lack of evidence on adequate settings of parameters and the need for intensive professional training to build experience enough to be able to set parameters in different clinical conditions.

Critical Perspectives on the Efficacy of HFCWO

Various ACT modalities, including IPV, may be used effectively, either alone or in combination. To date, however, there exists no criteria on the use of such modalities in children, regarding the opportunity and level of effectiveness. Therefore, other techniques, alone or in combination, may be required to clear secretions once mobilized centrally following intrapulmonary percussive ventilation. Further research is required to evaluate the safety and efficacy of HFCWO in the care of patients with CF. Highlights the recommendations from the authors of this state-of-the-art review for peripheral ACT's, considering all the evidence published since these guidelines and non-randomized controlled trials. Oscillatory devices are known to be very expensive, they are not readily available, and clinical or statistical evidence showed no significant differences.

Conclusion

High-Frequency Chest Wall Oscillation (HFCWO) emerges as a promising therapeutic approach for managing cystic fibrosis (CF) exacerbations in pediatrics. The technology offers potential advantages in secretion clearance and respiratory function improvement. However, challenges and controversies remain regarding HFCWO use. These include limited device availability and affordability in some regions, lack of standardized parameter settings for optimal application and the need for further research to definitively establish safety and efficacy in the CF population. Overall, HFCWO appears to be a promissory complementary technique in CF management while ongoing research is crucial for its optimization and its potential integration to other therapies in comprehensive care.

Key Messages

1. High-frequency chest wall oscillation (HFCWO) is an airway clearance technique by which external forces are applied to the chest through an inflatable vest connected to a device that generates vibrations at variable frequency and intensity [15].
2. Medical literature has shown the benefits of HFCWO in CF in children. The addition of HFCWO to medical treatment has proved to decrease airway obstruction and benefit individuals with cystic fibrosis during acute respiratory exacerbations.
3. Availability and cost of devices can be constraints. Lack of evidence on optimal configurations and the need for intensive training for professionals are noted as challenges.
4. The need for further research to evaluate the safety and efficacy of HFCWO in the care of CF patients is highlighted. Important to add, other techniques may be necessary to remove secretions once centrally mobilized.

References

[1] Warwick WJ, Hansen LG. The long-term effect of high-frequency chest compression therapy on pulmonary complications of cystic fibrosis. *Pediatric Pulmonology* 1991; 11(3):265-71.

[2] King, M., D. M. Phillips, D. Gross, V. Vartian, H. K. Chang, A. Zidulka, Enhanced tracheal mucus clearance with high-frequency chest wall compression. *Am Rev Respir Dis* 1983;128 (3) 511-515.

[3] Bidiwala A., Volpe L., Halaby C., Fazzari M., Valsamis C.., Pirzada M. A comparison of high-frequency chest wall oscillation and intrapulmonary percussive ventilation for airway clearance in pediatric patients with tracheostomy. *Postgrad Med* 2017. Mar;129(2):276-282.

[4] Kempainen R. R., Milla C., Dunitz J., et al. Comparison of settings used for high-frequency chest-wall compression in cystic fibrosis. *Respir Care* 2010;55(6):695-701.

[5] Leemans G., Belmans D., Van Holsbeke C., Becker B., Vissers D., Ides K., Verhulst S., Van Hoorenbeeck K. The effectiveness of a mobile high-frequency chest wall

oscillation (HFCWO) device for airway clearance. *Pediatr Pulmonol* 2020 Aug;55(8):1984-1992.

[6] McCarren B., Alison J. A. Physiological effects of vibration in subjects with cystic fibrosis. *Eur Respir J* 2006;27(6):1204-1209.

[7] Stanislav Krasovskij, Elena Amelina, Maria Usacheva, Victor Samoylenko, Natalia Krilova. *European Respiratory Journal Sep* 2013; 42 (Suppl 57).

[8] Main E., Rand S. Conventional chest physiotherapy compared to other airway clearance techniques for cystic fibrosis. *Cochrane Database Syst Rev* 2023; May 5;5(5).

[9] Wilson L. M., Saldanha I. J., Robinson K. A. Active cycle of breathing technique for cystic fibrosis. *Cochrane Database Syst Rev* 2023; Feb 2;2(2).

[10] Sontag M. K., Quittner A. L., Modi A. C., Koenig J. M., Giles D., Oermann C. M., et al. Lessons learned from a randomized trial of airway secretion clearance techniques in cystic fibrosis. *Pediatric Pulmonology* 2010;45(3):291-300.

[11] Modi A. C., Lim C. S., Yu N., Geller D., Wagner M. H., Quittner A. L. A multi-method assessment of treatment adherence for children with cystic fibrosis. *J Cyst Fibros* 2006;5(3):177-185.

[12] White T., Miller J., Smith G. L., McMahon W. M. Adherence and psycho-pathology in children and adolescents with cystic fibrosis. *Eur Child Adolesc Psychiatry* 2009;18(2):96-104.

[13] White D., Stiller K., Haensel N. Adherence of adult cystic fibrosis patients with airway clearance and exercise regimens. *J Cyst Fibros* 2007;6(3):163-170.

[14] Benoit C. M., Christensen E., Nickel A. J., Shogren S., Johnson M., Thompson E. F., McNamara J. Objective Measures of Vest Therapy Adherence Among Pediatric Subjects with Cystic Fibrosis. *Respir Care* 2020 Dec;65(12):1831-1837.

[15] Longhini F., Bruni A., Garofalo E., Ronco C., Gusmano A., Cammarota G., Pasin L., Frigerio P., Chiumello D., Navalesi P. Chest physiotherapy improves lung aeration in hyper secretive critically ill patients: a pilot randomized physiological study. *Crit Care* 2020 Aug 3;24(1):479.

Chapter 16

High-Frequency Chest Wall Oscillation Applications for Non-Cystic Fibrosis Children

Merve Erdem, MD
and Selman Kesici*, MD
Department of Pediatric Intensive Care Medicine, Life Support Center,
Hacettepe University Faculty of Medicine, Ankara, Turkiye

Abstract

This chapter emphasizes the anatomical and physiological differences between pediatric and adult respiratory systems, the importance of secretion clearance in children and the effectiveness of high-frequency chest wall oscillation (HFCWO) on secretion clearance in children. In this chapter, it was also explained how HFCWO works, its non-invasive nature and ability to improve pulmonary function by generating cough-like shear forces to enhance airway clearance. In addition, current chapter reviews the use of HFCWO in patients with chronic lung diseases, bronchiectasis, neuromuscular diseases, and those in intensive care settings.

Recent research indicates the potential benefits of HFCWO in infection prevention, enhanced airway clearance, and reduced hospitalizations, particularly in bronchiectasis and primary ciliary dyskinesia. In post-operative care, HFCWO has shown promising results, particularly in patients undergoing thoracic and upper abdominal surgery and lung transplantation.

High-frequency chest wall oscillation has traditionally been used for cystic fibrosis rehabilitation, but studies suggest potential for other

---

* Corresponding Author's Email: drselmankesici@gmail.com.

In: High-frequency Chest Wall Oscillation Therapy in Critical Ill Patients
Editor: Antonio M. Esquinas
ISBN: 979-8-89530-264-4
© 2025 Nova Science Publishers, Inc.

indications and children. HFCWO is an option to improve the quality of life for children in whom clearance of secretions is vital.

Keywords: children, critical care, chronic conditions, healthcare, respiratory disease

Introduction

The traditional saying, 'Children are not small adults,' which we have all been told many times in medical school, makes much sense for the respiratory system. Respiratory physiology is very different in young children, especially in neonates and infants, compared to adults [1]. Respiratory-related morbidity and mortality is a significant problem even in healthy children.

Children's airways are smaller and more prone to collapse, resulting in increased airway resistance and work of breathing. Babies breathe mainly through the nose in the early infant period, further increasing airway resistance. Having narrower airways creates a tendency for obstruction and collapse. Unlike the adult larynx, the pediatric larynx is anatomically narrowest at the subglottic level and functionally at the cricoid cartilage. Alveolarization of the distal airways occurs mainly after birth and continues until adolescence. The pediatric chest wall, especially in infants, has greater compliance and strong recoil, which increases the load on the diaphragm muscle. Neonates, infants and young children have a higher metabolic rate and oxygen demand. As a result, their resting oxygen consumption is more than double that of adults [1, 2]. Their higher oxygen demand and smaller functional residual capacity make them unable to tolerate rapid desaturation. Additionally, impaired respiratory defense mechanisms in children, such as mucociliary clearance in adenoid hypertrophy, lead to difficulties clearing secretions from the respiratory system, making them more prone to infections and complications [3]. Developmental changes in the respiratory system and immunologic and neurologic maturation, result in differences between children and adults in almost every respect [1, 2]. Clearing secretions is even more crucial in children than adults due to significant anatomical and physiological differences.

Medical advancements in recent years have unequivocally paved the way for revolutionary therapies that undeniably enhance the quality of life for patients suffering from respiratory conditions. High-frequency chest wall oscillation is one of the peripheral airway clearance techniques that has gained prominence. It has been initially recognized for its efficacy in treating individuals with cystic fibrosis (CF) [4, 5]. Numerous studies demonstrate that HFCWO effectively mobilizes airway secretions in various medical conditions (such as neuromuscular disorders) [6-8].

Secretion clearance in children with neuromuscular disorders; for an effective cough, taking a deep enough breath is crucial. For the intrathoracic pressure to increase, the glottis must close briefly, followed by forced air expulsion by an expulsive glottic opening with abdominal contraction [9]. Cough expiratory airflow is referred to as peak cough flow. Peak cough flow is impaired in individuals with glottic closure problems and weak or impaired inspiratory-expiratory muscles [4].

In neuromuscular diseases (NMD), weakness of the inspiratory muscles leads to a decrease in vital capacity and hypoventilation. Severe bulbar and glottic dysfunction leads to decreased coughing ability, secretion retention and progressive respiratory morbidity. Difficulty swallowing may lead to the accumulation of saliva and mucus in the vallecula and piriform sinuses. Excess secretions and ineffective coughing predispose to recurrent respiratory infections, which are the leading cause of morbidity and mortality in patients with NMD [4]. Adequate secretion clearance allows patients with NMD to live longer and to be ventilator-independent [4, 10].

Given the above, research suggests that HFCWO benefits children outside the CF spectrum [10]. This chapter delves into the potential applications and advantages of HFCWO in respiratory conditions.

Understanding High-Frequency Chest Wall Oscillation

Working Principle

High-frequency chest wall oscillation, a peripheral airway clearance technique, generates cough-like shear forces with transient increases in airflow at low lung volumes by applying sharp compression pulses with an air pulse generator and inflating vast [4, 11]. The goal is to move secretions from the smallest and deepest airways towards the larger airways (those branching off at the 12th generation of the bronchial tree and above). Applying HFCWO results in increased airflow and mucus, reduced mucus thickness, and higher cilia activity, the natural mechanisms for cleaning the airway [5, 11]. HFCWO achieves 300–1500 staccato coughs to move secretions with enhanced central and peripheral airway clearance [5]. There are mobile and immobile forms.

HFCWO can be administered every four hours in adult intensive care unit patients with mechanical ventilation (MV) [12]. Additionally, in patients dependent on MV, HFCWO can be administered without weaning them from the MV [4].

Advantages

High-frequency chest wall oscillation is non-invasive and does not require cooperation during its performance. High-frequency chest wall oscillation is a non-invasive airway clearance technique designed to mobilize and remove excess mucus from the respiratory tract [13]. Since HFCWO does not necessarily require patient cooperation, it can be used in infants, children, and even tracheostomy and/or bulbar failure or intellectual impairment [4].

This airway clearance technique enhances patients' quality of life by improving their pulmonary function. Nicolini et al. showed that HFCWO significantly improved parameters associated with bronchial obstruction (FVC, FEV1), dyspnea and patients' quality of life compared to conventional chest physiotherapy [14]. Hristara-Papadopoulou et al. suggest airway clearance techniques facilitate mucus removal while improving pulmonary function [15]. Longhini F. et al. observed a significant increase in functional residual capacity during HFCWO application [12].

Aa study by Ge J. et al. found that adults with severe craniocerebral injury, treated with tracheostomy and mechanical ventilation, showed better results during receiving HFCWO twice daily. This group exhibited improved oxygenation, increased lung static compliance and higher levels of surfactant proteins in the airways compared to those who received HFCWO once or not at all [16].

Disadvantages

High-frequency chest wall oscillation is a costly physiotherapy method, and certain limitations have been identified that restrict its use.

It is an expensive method compared to other airway clearance techniques. Its application is limited in the presence of indwelling catheters and chest tubes; hemodynamic instability and unstable head and neck injuries are contraindications [5, 10].

There are precautions when using it in patients with weakened cough reflexes.

In patients with neuromuscular diseases, the cough reflex is not strong enough, and swallowing dysfunction is present. HFCWO mobilize excessive amounts of the patient's secretions into the central airways, which the patient may not tolerate due to the conditions mentioned earlier. This situation may even cause the patient to respiratory arrest. Therefore, when using HFCWO in patients with NMD, equipment should be available to clear the airways of the mobilized secretions quickly [4].

Applications in Non-Cystic Fibrosis Children

Many studies about HFCWO involve adults with non-CF diseases. Studies on the use of HFCWO in children have been limited due to distrust of this technique and its high cost. In addition, many studies showed that it did not provide a significant difference compared to traditional chest physiotherapy. However, HFCWO has been used for a long time in patients of many different age groups to manage chronic conditions such as bronchiectasis and neuromuscular disorders [11].

In intensive care settings: Non-excreted airway secretions lead to transient mucociliary dysfunction. Intrapulmonary shunts develop, and tidal volume decreases. As a result, atelectasis, bronchopulmonary inflammation, pneumonia, respiratory arrest, and even death may occur [11]. There are many studies on the impact of HFCWO use on adult respiratory function. However, a comprehensive study on HFCWO usage in children is needed.

According to a study by Longhini F. et al. on adults, HFCWO should only be used on patients with excessive mucus secretion during mechanical ventilation. The researchers believed that this approach would help save time and reduce the workload for nurses and physiotherapists. However, traditional chest physiotherapy is just as effective for patients with normal mucus secretion during mechanical ventilation, and no additional benefits have been demonstrated [12].

Huang WC. et al. reported that the HFCWO has been an excellent choice for airway clearance in critically ill patients with prolonged intubation but has provided no extra benefit for weaning [17].

In adults, Kuyrukluyıldız U. et al. stated that combined techniques can prevent the development of pulmonary atelectasis or hospital-acquired pneumonia more than routine pulmonary rehabilitation, although HFCWO has costly equipment. HFCWO has not positively impact the length of intubation and stay in ICU [11].

Non-CF chronic lung diseases and bronchiectasis: HFCWO is beneficial in children with bronchiectasis, a condition characterized by irreversible dilation of bronchi. HFCWO helps to promote mucus clearance, which may, in turn, prevent recurrent infections and improve respiratory well-being.

A study by Barto TL. et al. demonstrated that hospitalizations and antibiotic use have decreased, and airway clearance has improved after HFCWO treatment in adults with non-cystic fibrosis bronchiectasis [18].

In a study by Gokdemir Y. et al. conventional pulmonary rehabilitation was compared to HFCWO in children with primary ciliary dyskinesia. The study found that both pulmonary rehabilitation methods resulted in a significant increase in pulmonary function tests, but there was no significant difference between the two methods. However, according to the study, HFCWO has been more comfortable for patients. Therefore, HFCWO is a suitable alternative for children with chronic lung disease who have low compliance with conventional pulmonary rehabilitation methods [19].

Neuromuscular diseases: Patients with neuromuscular diseases often have difficulty in clearing secretions due to impaired respiratory muscle function. HFCWO offers these patients a non-invasive way to support airway patency, potentially reducing the risk of respiratory complications [4, 20].

In a study by Lechtzin N. et al. in which most patients were children, total medical costs, hospitalizations and pneumonia episodes in patients with NMDs were shown to decrease after HFCWO administration. This study has recommended promoting HFCWO use in the routine care of children and adults with neuromuscular diseases [21].

Yuan et al. stated that high-frequency chest wall oscillation in children with NMD-cerebral palsy was safe, no side effects developed, and the need for hospitalization was reduced [10].

Keating JM et al. reported that a patient with spinal muscular atrophy type 1 did not benefit from increased ventilation pressure (non-invasive mechanical ventilator), manual percussion, and mechanical insufflation/exsufflation applied for airway clearance. However, ventilator-free time was extended with HFCWO, showing improved patient tolerance [22].

High-frequency chest wall oscillation has been shown to have no severe adverse effects on managing respiratory conditions in children with severe global developmental delays [23].

Postoperative care: There is no data on applying HFCWO in children for a post-op term, and there is little data on adults. Patients who have undergone thoracic and upper abdominal surgery experience challenges such as ineffective cough, decreased lung volume, and impaired airway clearance during the postoperative period, which lead to pulmonary complications. These complications, including atelectasis and pneumonia, are often attributed to impaired breathing due to chest expansion, coughing and post-operative pain. HFCWO has been shown to have acute effects on clearing secretions and reducing airway resistance, making it a valuable tool to overcome the challenges of the postoperative period. Thoracic compression associated with HFCWO significantly affects secretion removal and respiratory system impedance [24]. The use of HFCWO in lung transplantation has been investigated, indicating its potential role in facilitating the removal of secretions post-transplant [6].

Conclusion

While primarily recognized for cystic fibrosis treatment, HFCWO's potential benefits in children without CF are under exploration. Its non-invasive nature and efficacy in promoting airway clearance make it a promise for children with respiratory issues. As studies on HFCWO use have been increased, it might be integral in comprehensive respiratory care in selected patients. HFCWO's potential benefits in non-CF children, especially those with neuromuscular conditions, require further investigation for broader utilization and improved respiratory care.

Key Messages

1. Secretion clearance is critical in children because their respiratory system differs anatomically.
2. HFCWO improve respiratory function by enhancing secretion clearance in children.

3. HFCWO is a potential therapeutic modality for non-CF pediatric patients, highlighting its promising role in respiratory care.
4. Many studies suggest that HFCWO offers potential benefits for various conditions, including bronchiectasis and neuromuscular diseases.
5. HFCWO clears secretions in postoperative patients, particularly after thoracic and upper abdominal surgeries.
6. The use of HFCWO is limited by its cost.
7. Effective aspiration and emergency response equipment must be accessible when administering HFCWO to patients with weak cough reflexes.
8. HFCWO has limited applicability in children due to its non-cooperative nature.

References

[1] Di Cicco, M., Kantar, A., Masini, B., et al. Structural and functional development in airways throughout childhood: Children are not small adults. *Pediatric Pulmonology* 2021. 56(1): p. 240-251.

[2] Saikia, D. and B. Mahanta, Cardiovascular and respiratory physiology in children. *Indian journal of anaesthesia* 2019. 63(9): p. 690.

[3] Marusiakova, L., Durdik, P., Jesenak, M., et al. Ciliary beat frequency in children with adenoid hypertrophy. *Pediatric Pulmonology* 2020. 55(3): p. 666-673.

[4] Chatwin, M., Toussaint, M., Gonçalves, M. R., et al. Airway clearance techniques in neuromuscular disorders: a state of the art review. *Respiratory medicine* 2018. 136: p. 98-110.

[5] Chaudary, N. and G. Balasa, Airway clearance therapy in cystic fibrosis patients insights from a clinician providing cystic fibrosis care. *International journal of general medicine* 2021: p. 2513-2521.

[6] Esguerra-Gonzalez, A., Ilagan-Honorio, M., Fraschilla, S., et al. CNE article: pain after lung transplant: high-frequency chest wall oscillation vs chest physiotherapy. *American journal of critical care* 2013. 22(2): p. 115-124.

[7] de Alvarenga, G. M., Remigio Gamba, H., Elisa Hellman, L., et al. Physiotherapy intervention during level I of pulmonary rehabilitation on chronic obstructive pulmonary disease: a systematic review. *The open respiratory medicine journal* 2016. 10: p. 12.

[8] Huang, H. P., Chen, K, C., Tsai, C. L., et al. Effects of High-Frequency Chest Wall Oscillation on Acute Exacerbation of Chronic Obstructive Pulmonary Disease: A Systematic Review and Meta-Analysis of Randomized Controlled Trials. *International Journal of Chronic Obstructive Pulmonary Disease* 2022: p. 2857-2869.

[9] Leith D E. The development of cough. *American Review of Respiratory Disease* 1985. 131(S5): p. S39-S42.
[10] Yuan N. et al. Safety, tolerability, and efficacy of high-frequency chest wall oscillation in pediatric patients with cerebral palsy and neuromuscular diseases: an exploratory randomized controlled trial. *Journal of child neurology* 2010. 25(7): p. 815-821.
[11] Kuyrukluyildiz, U., Binici, O., Kupeli, İ., et al. What is the best pulmonary physiotherapy method in ICU? *Canadian Respiratory Journal* 2016:2016:4752467.
[12] Longhini F., Bruni, A., Garofalo, E., et al. Chest physiotherapy improves lung aeration in hypersecretive critically ill patients: a pilot randomized physiological study. *Critical Care* 2020. 24: p. 1-10.
[13] Mahajan A. K., Diette, G. B., Hatipoğlu, U., et al. High-frequency chest wall oscillation for asthma and chronic obstructive pulmonary disease exacerbations: a randomized sham-controlled clinical trial. *Respiratory research* 2011. 12: p. 1-7.
[14] Nicolini, A., Cardini, F., Landucci, N., et al. Effectiveness of treatment with high-frequency chest wall oscillation in patients with bronchiectasis. *BMC Pulmonary medicine* 2013. 13(1): p. 1-8.
[15] Hristara-Papadopoulou A., Tsanakas, J., Diomou, G., et al. Current devices of respiratory physiotherapy. Hippokratia 2008. 12(4): p. 211.
[16] Ge, J., Ye, Y., Tan, Y., et al. High-frequency chest wall oscillation multiple times daily can better reduce the loss of pulmonary surfactant and improve lung compliance in mechanically ventilated patients. *Heart & Lung* 2023. 61: p. 114-119.
[17] Huang, W., Wu, P., Chen, C., et al. High-frequency chest wall oscillation in prolonged mechanical ventilation patients: a randomized controlled trial. *The Clinical Respiratory Journal* 2016. 10(3): p. 272-281.
[18] Barto, T. L., Maselli, D. J., Daignault, S., et al. Real-life experience with high-frequency chest wall oscillation vest therapy in adults with non-cystic fibrosis bronchiectasis. *Ther Adv Respir Dis* 2020; 14: 1753466620932508.
[19] Gokdemir, Y., Karadag-Saygi, E., Erdem, E., et al. Comparison of conventional pulmonary rehabilitation and high-frequency chest wall oscillation in primary ciliary dyskinesia. *Pediatric pulmonology* 2014. 49(6): p. 611-616.
[20] Giacomino, K., Hilfiker, R., Magnin, T., et al. A systematic review on the effects of high-frequency chest wall compression and intrapulmonary percussive ventilation in patients with neuromuscular disease. F1000Research, 2022. 10: p. 10.
[21] Lechtzin N, Wolfe L F, and Frick K D. The impact of high-frequency chest wall oscillation on healthcare use in patients with neuromuscular diseases. *Annals of the American Thoracic Society* 2016. 13(6): p. 904-909.
[22] Keating, J. M., Collins, N., Bush, A., et al. High-frequency chest-wall oscillation in a noninvasive-ventilation-dependent patient with type 1 spinal muscular atrophy. *Respiratory care* 2011. 56(11): p. 1840-1843.
[23] Winfield, N. R., Barker, N. J., Turner, E. R., et al. Non-pharmaceutical management of respiratory morbidity in children with severe global developmental delay. *Cochrane Database of Systematic Reviews* 2014(10).

[24] Strickland, S. L., Rubin, B. K., Drescher, G. S., et al. AARC clinical practice guideline: effectiveness of nonpharmacologic airway clearance therapies in hospitalized patients. *Respiratory care* 2013. 58(12): p. 2187-2193.

About the Editor

Antonio M. Esquinas, MD, PhD is a Physician of the ICU of Hospital Morales Meseguer (Murcia, Spain), FCCP, FNIV, Member of the Respiratory NIV Group in ERS since 2009, and Member of the ERS College of Experts.

Dr. Esquinas has developed scientific teaching activities and publications focusing on NIV-acute and chronic respiratory failure. He has over 242 chapters, 552 articles, and 69 edited books edited to his credit.

Further, Dr. Esquinas is the Founder of the International School of NIV (2008), International Association, Academy and College of NIV and Ibero American Association of Bioethics in NIV.

Regarding his trajectory as researcher in the field of NIV, Dr. Esquinas was a visiting researcher at Anaesthesiology Policlinico Umberto I (1999, Rome), Fondazione Salvatore Maugeri (FSM) (Florence, 2000), FSM-Pneumology Department, Brescia (1999), Slovakian Institute-Pneumology Kosice, Slovakia (2011) and ICU-Gemelli Hospital (2012, 2013, Italy).

His main research interests are aimed at establishing clinical analysis and predictive models for NIV in hypoxemic- hypercapnic, NIV-difficult weaning, chronic critically ill patients, novel ventilatory approaches and epidemiological analysis of NIV use.

Dr. Esquinas hopes this book will accessibly contribute to emerging groups and offer platforms for younger researchers who want to develop a scientific career in non-invasive ventilatory approaches.

ORCID iD:
https://orcid.org/0000-0003-0571-2050

Google Scholar:
https://scholar.google.es/citations?user=uyhKxeAAAAAJ&hl=es

ResearchGate:
https://www.researchgate.net/profile/Antonio-Esquinas

PubMed:
https://pubmed.ncbi.nlm.nih.gov/?term=esquinas+a&sort=date&size=100

Books:
https://www.amazon.com/-/es/stores/author/B08G2MG7PW

Index

A

Acapella, 30
Acute Physiology and Chronic Health Evaluation II (APACHE II), 95
acute respiratory ailments, 1, 4
aerosolized medications, 125
air-mucus interaction, 7, 8, 11, 12
airway clearance, 2, 6, 7, 8, 12, 13, 15, 16, 17, 18, 19, 25, 26, 29, 30, 31, 33, 34, 35, 38, 40, 41, 42, 45, 49, 50, 51, 52, 53, 54, 55, 56, 60, 61, 62, 65, 70, 71, 72, 81, 86, 87, 88, 89, 91, 98, 106, 113, 115, 118, 121, 122, 123, 124, 125, 127, 129, 130, 131, 132, 133,134, 139, 146, 149, 152, 153, 155, 156, 157, 158, 159, 160, 161, 162, 164
airway clearance device(s), 16, 19, 25, 35
airway clearance technique(s) (ACT), 7, 8, 12, 15, 23, 30, 33, 35, 38, 40, 41, 42, 45, 52, 54, 55, 71, 88, 106, 113, 115, 122, 127, 128, 129, 130, 131, 133, 134, 139, 145, 146, 151, 152, 153, 156, 157, 158, 162
airway mucus clearance, 43, 44
airway obstruction, 40, 43, 95, 121, 123, 146, 149, 152
airway secretions, 2, 54, 61, 76, 98, 102, 118, 124, 126, 137, 139, 140, 157, 159
airway secretions devices, 102, 118
airways, 2, 4, 7, 8, 9, 10, 11, 12, 13, 17, 24, 32, 38, 41, 43, 44, 54, 63, 65, 67, 68, 69, 76, 102, 104, 106, 109, 112, 123, 127, 129, 130, 137, 141, 147, 148, 156, 157, 158, 159, 162
alveolar ventilation, 12, 45, 122, 131, 132
Amyotrophic Lateral Sclerosis (ALS), 3, 5, 29, 30, 122, 124, 126, 128, 133, 134
antibiotics, 44, 65, 88, 104, 113, 115, 118, 136, 137, 138, 150
assisted airway clearance devices, 16
asymmetric oscillatory flow, 10

B

body mass index, 95, 111, 114
Breathlessness, Cough, and Sputum Scale (BCSS), 45, 47, 112
bronchiectasis, 2, 3, 4, 6, 16, 29, 30, 33, 35, 39, 40, 41, 44, 48, 49, 54, 65, 68, 77, 88, 89, 105, 108, 109, 110, 114, 115, 118, 119, 135, 141, 143, 147, 155, 159, 160, 162, 163
bronchoalveolar lavage (BAL), 137
bronchopulmonary hygiene techniques, 110

C

cardiovascular factors, 83
cerebral palsy, 121, 123, 134, 149, 160, 163
chest physical therapy, 2, 34, 37, 41, 43, 53, 54, 61, 63, 64, 122, 124, 128, 132
chest physical therapy (CPT), 2, 3, 17, 21, 34, 37, 41, 43, 53, 54, 61, 63, 64, 122, 124, 128, 132, 140
chest physical therapy and postural drainage (CPT/PD), 2
chest physiotherapy, 1, 3, 6, 13, 16, 39, 44, 45, 49, 52, 58, 61, 87, 88, 109, 112, 114,

118, 128, 140, 145, 146, 149, 153, 158, 159, 162, 163
chest wall vibration, 8, 9, 11, 13
chest X-ray, 46, 59, 61
children, 4, 6, 33, 34, 38, 40, 45, 49, 64, 125, 126, 129, 130, 133, 145, 146, 149, 150, 151, 152, 153, 155, 156, 157, 158, 159, 160, 161, 162, 163
chronic conditions, 98, 156, 159
chronic obstructive pulmonary disease (COPD), 1, 2, 3, 4, 5, 9, 16, 18, 29, 30, 31, 33, 39, 40, 42, 45, 48, 49, 68, 71, 72, 73, 77, 82, 84, 88, 91, 92, 95, 101, 102, 103, 104, 105, 110, 111, 112, 114, 115, 116, 117, 118, 119, 138, 141, 143, 162, 163
ciliary beat frequency, 44, 77, 162
community-acquired pneumonia (CAP), 4, 6
complex neuromuscular disorders (cNMD), 121, 123, 125
conventional chest physical therapy (CCPT), 47, 48, 53, 59, 61, 91, 118, 134, 139, 140, 145, 146, 150
cough augmentation strategies, 53
cough severity, 4
critical care, 1, 6, 67, 70, 72, 76, 80, 81, 90, 98, 101, 117, 119, 156, 162, 163
critically ill, 4, 6, 52, 61, 63, 71, 98, 99, 136, 153, 159, 163, 165
cystic fibrosis (CF), 1, 2, 3, 4, 5, 13, 14, 16, 18, 26, 29, 30, 33, 35, 38, 39, 40, 41, 42, 43, 44, 48, 49, 50, 54, 68, 69, 71, 72, 81, 87, 88, 89, 91, 105, 106, 108, 109, 115, 118, 133, 134, 135, 140, 141, 145, 146, 147, 148, 149, 151, 152, 153, 155, 157, 159, 160, 161,162

D

diaphragm dysfunction, 96
diaphragmatic thickening, 96
dyspnea, 3, 9, 39, 68, 88, 103, 104, 111, 112, 113, 114, 123, 141, 158

E

endotracheal tubes, 47, 51, 59, 68, 136, 140
exacerbations, 3, 5, 45, 65, 69, 70, 71, 73, 89, 92, 101, 102, 104, 112, 117, 118, 119, 141, 145, 146, 148, 149, 150, 151, 152, 163
expectorants, 53
extubation, 46, 52, 59, 68, 71, 77, 87, 93, 94, 95, 97, 98, 99, 139
extubation failure, 52, 68, 93, 95, 97, 98, 99

F

fiberoptic bronchoscope, 2
flow oscillation, 10, 12, 86
flutter, 30, 44
flutter devices, 44
forced expiratory volume in first second (FEV$_1$), 40, 45, 46, 47, 82, 87, 89, 103, 113, 114, 150, 158
forced vibrations, 9
forced vital capacity (FVC), 3, 39, 40, 45, 46, 47, 82, 87, 89, 103, 111, 112, 114, 128, 150, 158
functional residual capacity (FRC), 11, 30, 45, 126, 156, 158

H

healthcare, 31, 35, 38, 70, 72, 73, 81, 87, 90, 104, 109, 123, 124, 128, 133, 137, 156, 163
heart failure, 83, 95, 104
high-flow nasal cannula therapy (HFNC), 75, 76, 77, 78, 79, 97, 105
high-frequency chest wall compression (HFCC), 2, 5, 13, 15, 16, 17, 18, 19, 20, 21, 22, 23, 24, 25, 27, 30, 49, 53, 54, 81, 82, 85, 89, 91, 124, 127, 128, 133, 146, 147, 150, 152, 163
high-frequency chest wall oscillation (HFCWO), 1, 2, 3, 4, 5, 6, 7, 13, 14, 15, 16, 17, 19, 25, 26, 29, 30, 31, 33, 34, 35, 37, 38, 39, 40, 41, 42, 43, 44, 45, 46, 47,

48, 49, 50, 51, 52, 53, 54, 55, 59, 61, 62, 63, 64, 65, 66, 67, 68, 69, 70, 71, 72, 73, 75, 76, 78, 79, 80, 81, 82, 85, 86, 87, 88, 89, 90, 91, 92, 93, 98, 101, 102, 106, 107, 108, 109, 110, 111, 112, 113, 114, 115, 116, 118, 119, 121, 122, 124, 125, 127, 128, 129, 132, 133, 134, 135, 136, 139, 140, 141, 142, 143, 145, 146, 147, 148, 149, 150, 151, 152, 153, 155, 156, 157, 158, 159, 160, 161, 162, 163
high-frequency chest wall oscillation devices, 16
hospital-acquired infections, 136
hospital-acquired pneumonia (HAP), 68, 135, 136, 138, 141, 142, 160
hospitalizations, 3, 44, 45, 65, 88, 89, 123, 125, 145, 148, 155, 160
hypercapnia, 94, 95, 105, 123, 133
hypersecretion, 3, 12, 111, 116, 119, 124
hypothyroidism, 84
hypoventilation, 123, 157

I

infection, 44, 53, 64, 65, 71, 75, 77, 101, 102, 104, 109, 114, 121, 123, 125, 126, 127, 136, 137, 139, 155
inflammation, 3, 52, 53, 65, 69, 104, 119, 125, 126, 141, 147, 159
inspiratory muscles, 115, 121, 123, 126, 157
intensive care unit(s) (ICUs), 4, 39, 40, 41, 47, 49, 57, 58, 60, 61, 72, 73, 75, 77, 78, 79, 87, 90, 93, 94, 95, 98, 99, 101, 136, 137, 138, 139, 141, 142, 158, 160, 163, 165
interactions, 10, 11, 12, 52, 55, 60, 65, 83
intrapulmonary percussive ventilation (IPPV), 16, 29, 30, 42, 119, 122, 124, 127, 129, 130, 132, 151, 152, 163
intubation, 46, 52, 59, 68, 75, 76, 77, 78, 79, 84, 95, 105, 136, 137, 138, 139, 140, 159, 160
invasive mechanical ventilation, 39, 46, 67, 72, 96, 135, 136, 139, 141, 142

ischemia, 83

L

left ventricular end diastolic pressure (LVEDP), 82, 83
lung flute, 30
lung function, 1, 3, 39, 40, 44, 65, 69, 71, 76, 77, 104, 111, 112, 116, 117, 118, 123, 133, 141, 145, 148, 149, 150
lungs, 4, 8, 10, 11, 20, 21, 22, 24, 25, 29, 30, 31, 43, 65, 67, 69, 82, 108, 114, 121, 123, 124, 126, 137, 140, 146, 147, 148

M

mechanical insufflation-exsufflation, 53, 87, 127
mechanical ventilation, 26, 39, 41, 46, 47, 49, 51, 52, 53, 54, 56, 57, 58, 59, 61, 62, 63, 67, 68, 73, 76, 81, 82, 90, 91, 94, 95, 97, 98, 99, 105, 134, 135, 136, 138, 139, 140, 141, 142, 158, 159
mechanical ventilator, 26, 39, 46, 52, 55, 56, 59, 60, 81, 118, 160
mechanical vibrations, 9, 11
metabolic factors, 83, 84
morbidity, 43, 63, 65, 71, 93, 95, 121, 122, 123, 124, 135, 136, 137, 141, 156, 157, 163
mortality, 43, 53, 63, 65, 71, 76, 85, 87, 93, 94, 95, 103, 105, 106, 117, 122, 123, 124, 134, 135, 136, 137, 141, 156, 157
mucoactive therapies, 53
mucociliary clearance (MCC), 4, 11, 12, 25, 52, 61, 75, 77, 78, 79, 102, 106, 115, 118, 122, 125, 126, 136, 145, 146, 156
mucociliary clearance impairment, 122, 125
mucociliary transport, 8, 13, 77, 142, 147
mucociliary transport system, 77
mucolytics, 53
mucus clearance, 1, 2, 4, 9, 11, 13, 21, 49, 53, 55, 56, 58, 61, 65, 73, 102, 105, 106, 109, 125, 126, 129, 160
mucus movement, 7, 17, 30, 56

mucus secretion, 33, 37, 43, 55, 109, 159

N

neurological diseases, 1, 3
neuromuscular diseases (NMDs), 2, 4, 18, 35, 38, 43, 44, 48, 73, 108, 115, 122, 123, 124, 125, 126, 127, 128, 129, 130, 131, 132, 133, 134, 155, 157, 159, 160, 162, 163
non-cystic fibrosis bronchiectasis, 43, 49, 73, 92, 119, 160, 163
nutritional factors, 84

O

oscillating pressure, 11, 37, 39, 41
oscillation frequency, 51, 58, 61, 65, 116
oscillation(s), 2, 5, 7, 8, 9, 11, 12, 13, 17, 24, 25, 26, 31, 33, 34, 38, 39, 40, 41, 46, 47, 49, 51, 54, 55, 56, 58, 60, 61, 65, 72, 80, 82, 89, 91, 102, 106, 107, 108, 109, 110, 111, 112, 116, 118, 119, 128, 130, 133, 134, 146, 147, 148, 149, 158, 163
oscillatory clearance index (OCI), 130
oscillatory positive expiratory pressure, 53
oxygen therapy, 75, 76, 77, 79, 97, 101, 102, 104, 105
oxygenation, 1, 4, 40, 46, 57, 67, 72, 75, 76, 78, 94, 97, 105, 106, 109, 112, 115, 126, 137, 149, 158

P

patient adherence, 3, 72, 111
patient-ventilator asynchrony, 57, 61
peak expiratory flow rate(s) (PEFR), 3, 39, 46
pediatric, 1, 4, 5, 6, 69, 71, 72, 80, 133, 134, 145, 146, 152, 153, 155, 156, 162, 163
pendelluft, 11, 12
percussive waveforms, 19
pharmacological therapy, 102, 104, 112
physiotherapy, 3, 13, 39, 53, 73, 87, 101, 102, 103, 106, 108, 109, 114, 115, 116, 127, 128, 133, 134, 146, 150, 158, 162, 163
physiotherapy techniques, 106, 146
pneumatic vest, 2, 44
pneumonia, 1, 4, 39, 40, 46, 53, 57, 64, 68, 70, 71, 87, 106, 113, 114, 115, 119, 124, 135, 136, 137, 138, 140, 141, 159, 160, 161
positive end-expiratory pressure (PEEP), 76, 97, 110, 116, 118
positive expiratory pressure (PEP), 5, 14, 42, 48, 50, 118, 129, 145, 146
postextubation respiratory failure, 94, 98
post-lung transplant care, 1, 3, 4
predictors, 93, 94
pressure settings, 15, 39, 56, 57, 58, 61
pressure waveforms, 17, 19, 20, 22
prevention, 68, 69, 71, 97, 98, 99, 103, 135, 136, 137, 138, 139, 140, 142, 155
prolonged mechanical ventilation (PMV), 46, 49, 51, 59, 62, 67, 68, 72, 73, 80, 91, 95, 135, 141, 163
psychological factors, 84
pulmonary edema, 83
pulmonary function tests, 39, 46, 112, 115, 160
pulmonary rehabilitation (PR), 7, 10, 46, 68, 72, 81, 82, 88, 89, 90, 91, 92, 105, 160, 162, 163
pulse generator, 19, 20, 25, 31, 32, 38, 63, 64, 148, 157

Q

quake, 30
quality of life, 40, 45, 47, 65, 70, 71, 88, 102, 104, 112, 114, 116, 118, 126, 141, 145, 146, 148, 150, 156, 158

R

respiratory disease, 5, 49, 71, 73, 88, 89, 106, 118, 119, 156, 163
respiratory factors, 84
respiratory functions, 1, 4, 110

Index

respiratory health, 1, 2, 64, 69, 70, 71, 125, 129, 132, 141, 149
respiratory infections, 44, 69, 77, 105, 126, 157
respiratory muscle capacity, 95
respiratory muscle weakness, 84, 121, 122, 123, 124, 137
respiratory secretions, 77, 95, 122, 123, 124, 132
respiratory system, 7, 9, 13, 65, 82, 122, 147, 155, 156, 161
respiratory therapy, 1, 2, 72, 115, 134, 139
rheological properties, 8, 12, 44, 125, 134

S

secretion removal, 29, 161
shortness of breath, 9, 88, 89, 141
sine wave, 20, 21, 22, 23, 24, 25, 54
spinal cord injuries (SCI), 124
spinal muscular atrophies (SMA), 122, 124, 126
spontaneous breathing trial (SBT), 82, 85, 94, 95, 96, 97, 99, 139, 140
sputum, 3, 4, 10, 22, 26, 38, 44, 45, 46, 47, 48, 52, 59, 60, 61, 89, 103, 104, 110, 111, 112, 113, 114, 115, 116, 126, 136, 137, 150
sputum clearance, 52, 61, 110
sputum expectoration, 45, 47, 136

T

tachycardia, 104
tachypnea, 104

tracheal mucus clearance, 1, 2, 5, 108, 118, 128, 134, 152
tracheal mucus clearance rate (TMCR), 2
tracheostomy(ies), 67, 93, 95, 130, 135, 136, 152, 158
triangle wave, 20, 21, 22, 23, 24, 25, 27

U

ultrasound, 96, 99

V

ventilator dependence, 82, 83, 84, 85
ventilator-associated pneumonia (VAP), 52, 69, 70, 71, 135, 136, 137, 138, 141, 142
Vest® Airway Clearance System, 59
vibration(s), iii, 7, 8, 9, 10, 11, 12, 13, 17, 30, 32, 38, 64, 65, 78, 106, 107, 127, 130, 148, 149, 152, 153
vital capacity (VC), 39, 82, 89, 112, 121, 123, 126, 130, 131, 157

W

waveforms, 15, 16, 19, 20, 21, 22, 24, 25, 26, 27, 55
weaning, 46, 51, 53, 59, 67, 70, 71, 73, 81, 83, 85, 87, 90, 91, 93, 94, 95, 96, 98, 99, 139, 158, 159, 165
weaning-induced cardiac dysfunction, 83, 90
work of breathing (WOB), 82, 83, 84, 95, 105, 123, 128, 156